EAT YOURSELF SKINNY 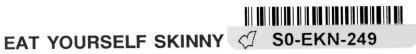 S0-EKN-249

Recipes and Menus by: PAMELA PLACE

The Diet Philosophy by: KEN PLACE

Published by:

PAMELA PRESS
2804 E. 30th Avenue
Spokane, WA 99223

EAT YOURSELF SKINNY

A Diet Plan and Recipe Collection
For Losing Weight and Keeping It Off

FOREWARD
==========

I lost 560 pounds and you can do it too.   Maybe you've already lost that much weight the same way I did. It's really pretty easy . . . just lose ten pounds every time you go on a diet. Gain it back, then six months later do it again. An average of ten pounds lost twice a year, for 28 years since college days is, sure enough, 560 pounds.

I always wanted to maintain my graduation weight of 165 pounds, which is acceptable for a 5'9" adult male with a stocky build. Call it a post-graduate goal. Then, with accounting degree in hand, I entered one of the most sedentary of occupations and in less than a year ballooned up to 185 pounds.

Twenty pounds overweight has been the average most of my adult life. About twice a year I got motivated and tried whichever diet was in vogue at the time and which seemed to fit my lifestyle. Typically I would stay on the diet for a few weeks and lose about ten pounds. I would gradually revert to my old eating habits and soon be carrying those pounds again, along with a few more picked up along the way. At one point I bulked up to 195 pounds.

I finally woke up to the fact that in order to keep weight off I needed A DIET TO LIVE WITH year in and year out. Short-term diet binges failed me, as they have failed millions of others.

During the past eight or ten years I have become increasingly aware of the health aspects of the food I eat and the potential harm to my body from ingesting the wrong foods to obtain some short-term weight loss. The answer for everyone is to EAT RIGHT FOR LIFE.

In 1987 I met the author when we were both single. Men (especially me) admired her figure and women envied it. No surplus fat. Still she never seemed to be on a diet. One of the lucky ones, right? Not really . . . just one of the smart ones.

She let me know there was no room for "fatties" in her life, but offered to put me on a diet that I could live with. She assured me I wouldn't feel hungry or weak . . . plenty of food, but – the right kind.

Now I am living proof that her method works. By following the common sense philosophies in this book and by eating food prepared by her recipes IT CAN WORK FOR YOU as well.

Seven weeks after I started eating Pamela's cooking, prepared from recipes in this book, I had lost 20 pounds and felt stronger than ever. Never before had I been able to continue on a diet for that long. Certainly I never lost that much weight before.

We were married on my 50th birthday and the weight is still off. Now my weight varies between 162 and 165 pounds. It's no problem maintaining that weight since I can stay on the diet because the food I eat is delicious, healthful and satisfying. Being a person who loves to eat, I really appreciate not feeling deprived of the food I love.

Having lived a life of fighting obesity, I sympathize with the millions of people in our society who want to lose weight and keep it off.

I asked Pamela to put together a collection of her delicious recipes and organize them into a book that can be shared with anyone interested in LIVING A HEALTHIER AND SLIMMER LIFE. The pages that follow are that result.

—— Kenneth T. Place
December, 1988

TABLE OF CONTENTS

THE DIET PHILOSOPHY

THE RECIPE SECTION

THE WIN – WIN – WIN WAY TO EAT

Going on a diet to lose weight doesn't mean you have to lose in other ways as well. You don't have to feel weak or hungry. You don't have to subject your bodily functions to the intake of harmful foods or to starvation. The philosophy underlying this book, along with the recipes and cooking methods which follow, avoids those unwanted forms of loss and REWARDS YOU WITH WINS instead.

The first way you win with this diet is by AVOIDING HARMFUL FOODS and thereby promoting an improvement in your personal health. Much research has been done by others in the field of nutrition and the effects of certain foods on the human body. This book is not intended to be a technical manual in this field, but rather, makes a common sense application of the knowledge gained through that research.

The next way you win is by INCREASING YOUR ENERGY LEVEL. The foods used in the following recipes are rich in good slow–burning carbohydrates which have the effect of giving you a steady energy level for a longer period of time. You will be eating those "good" foods, while at the same time you will be avoiding the kind of food that gives you the heavy, stuffed feeling after eating or, like sugars and other fast–burning carbohydrates, gives you a short–term energy burst but which soon leaves you hungry.

With the philosophy of eating and the recipes in this book there is another way you win, which may seem unimportant to some people, but which is very important to those of us who love to eat. It is the fact that YOU ARE NOT HUNGRY all of the time as you are with many diets. This is especially important because hunger and lack of satifying food, will cause a dieter to cheat and eventually go off most diets, resulting in yet another failed weight loss program. The fulfillment factor, probably more than any other, is the reason this diet is one you can live with year in and year out and thereby keep the weight off indefinitely once you have lost it.

The recipes in this book use ingredients which are available in most supermarkets. There are no expensive "plans" to buy. Likewise there are no health store items, no pills, powders or liquid "diets". Because of the emphasis on fruit, vegetables and grain products and the minimum of meats and other oily foods, you will probably experience LOWER FOOD COSTS for these recipes than what you are used to, so you win again.

SAY GOODBYE TO FORMER FRIENDS

==================================

"Farewell, Fats . . . "

A principal aim of the recipes in this book is to greatly reduce the amount of fats eaten. Ounce for ounce, fats are tops in calorie content among all foods. If we reduce fats in our diet it will naturally help us lose weight. Even if weight loss were not enough, there are very compelling health reasons as well, for cutting down on fats.

There is one detrimental effect on the blood caused by all fats, whether saturated or unsaturated. That effect is the formation of a fatty film around elements in the blood, which reduces its capacity for delivering oxygen to the body tissues. This "suffocation" can reduce the efficiency of the circulatory system by 5% to 20%, which explains why many people get sleepy after eating. The drowsiness signal comes from the brain, which is very sensitive to reductions in the amount of oxygen carried to it by the blood.

It is estimated that on an average, Americans consume 40% to 45% of their calories in the form of fats. Our goal with these recipes is to bring that down into the 5% to 10% range. You don't need to eat fatty foods to get enough fat in your diet to be healthy. All foods have at least some fat in them. In fact, a diet of fruit, grains and vegetables will contain 5% to 10% fat content in the calories eaten.

Much has been said by researchers about the effects of fats on raising the cholesterol level in the blood stream, thus contributing to atherosclerosis. Many fatty foods also increase the uric acid in body tissues and contribute to gout. If those unhealthy facts weren't bad enough, consider that fats in the blood can reduce the body's ability to metabolize, or burn off, carbohydrates. This in turn can eventually lead to a diabetic condition.

The American taste buds and appetite are most often satisfied by fats. People eat what they like, or what they are used to tasting, to get that satisfaction. The recipes in this book provide a way to change unhealthy eating habits by replacing high-calorie fatty foods with healthy foods properly seasoned. This in turn will provide the satisfaction needed for weight and health conscious people to continue eating right for life.

"So long, Sugar . . . "

The only thing we ever got from that false friend was some satisfaction for our sweet tooth. There is nothing else good about sugar, but plenty of bad. Mostly it makes us fat! It also contributes to increased levels of triglycerides in our blood and instability in our bloodsugar levels.

Sugar may also be one of the villians contributing to atherosclerosis by raising the level of fat and cholesterol in the blood stream. This happens when sugar, a simple carbohydrate, is not burned off but instead is converted into fat cells, thereby adding to the problems which come from too much fat in the blood.

About one–fourth of the sugar we eat comes "out of the bowl" and the other three–fourths comes as part of the ingredients of processed foods. That is why it is so important to read the label before deciding to purchase any food. Sugar is a highly concentrated food substance which has been robbed of any fiber or other nutrition and should be avoided as much as possible.

It doesn't really matter what form they come in, simple carbohydrates such as sugar, honey, molasses, corn syrup, dextrose, fructose, etc. all require virtually no digestion and rush directly into the bloodstream, then quickly burn off or convert to fat. Don't be fooled by brown sugar, which is table sugar with caramel coloring added. Likewise, "raw" sugar, merely includes small amounts of sugar cane fiber or sugar beet pulp in order to give it the taste of real raw sugar.

The recipes in this book replace sugar with either fruit juices or sugar substitutes. Once your sweet tooth adjusts to not having sugar in the diet you will find you don't need it for satisfaction. Soon, foods with regular sugars in them will seem too sweet. While complex carbohydrates will signal your appetite when you've had enough, you can never really be satisfied with sugar. But . . . you can be fat.

"Sayonara, Ol' Salt . . . "

For more than 50 years researchers have known that salt is a big contributor to hypertension, or high blood pressure. They are not sure just how salt creates hypertension, but they do know it changes the body's natural balance between water and salt. A small amount of salt added to your diet can cause your body to hold extra pounds of water to make up for the imbalance.

Extra water in your body causes your heart to work harder, because tissue between the blood capillaries is more tightly filled. This causes extra pressure between the vessel walls and interferes with the transfer of blood oxygen by the capillaries. Continued oxygen shortage can lead to circulation problems, arthritis, and stiffness in joints and muscles.

The taste of salt is something Americans crave in their diets much like they crave fats. That's why they eat an average of six to sixteen grams of salt per day, whereas our goal should be to reduce that daily intake to about four grams, or roughly one-half teaspoon.

Our body gets all of the salt it needs from the food we eat, so it does not need to be added out of necessity for our bodily functions. The recipes in this book do not include any added salt, and none should be used at the table. So, get rid of that salt shaker and help remove the temptation.

You will find these recipes use various methods of flavoring, including salt substitute, which make them delicious without requiring added salt. If you want to lose weight, you will be surprised how much less bulk you carry once you cut down on the salt in your daily diet.

"Beat it, Eggs . . . "

Besides the goal of losing weight by eating according to the recipes in this book, we are equally concerned about eating for health. That brings us back to our old nemesis, cholesterol. Controlling the cholesterol level in our bloodstream is so important we have to turn against our former friend, the egg.

It is a shame to give up on eggs because they are relatively low in fat, high in protein and full of minerals and vitamins. They are easy to use in cooking, inexpensive, long-lasting and have been a proven staple food for centuries. Their main flaw is the high cholesterol content in the yoke of the egg. But this flaw is a fatal one, so whole eggs have been eliminated from the recipes in this book.

In recipes which do require eggs, egg substitutes are used. Eggless foods are specified in cases where part of the ingredients include prepared items, such as noodles. The egg substitutes contain no fat, no cholesterol and are very low in calories.

The exception to the "no eggs" rule is the use of egg whites. If you do not have egg substitute on hand, it is acceptable to remove the yoke from the egg then use two egg whites to equal the same quantity as one whole egg. Several of the recipes in this book will use this alternate method.

The food color will be more pale when you use only the egg whites, but it will still taste delicious because of other flavoring techniques used. Keep in mind that the overriding benefit to eliminating eggs, or more specifically egg yokes, is the reduction in your cholesterol intake.

HERBS AND SPICES TO THE RESCUE

Until you try it, you may not believe you can make food taste good or be satisfying without using salt, sugar and oils. The fact that you can, however, is one of the basic premises of this entire book. It is time to expand your inventory of spices and learn just how valuable they are as replacements for the harmful ingredients you've been using for flavor.

The recipes in this book help you in your discovery of using herbs and spices. Once you develop more confidence in the use of these ingredients, try some experiments. For instance, if you like a sweeter taste use some coriander, ginger, cinnamon, nutmeg, allspice, curry, mace, cloves, mint or cardamom.

If you like stronger flavors experiment with garlic, oregano, basil, chives, sage, onion powder, bay leaves, thyme, parsley, dillweed, cumin, black pepper, mustard, rosemary or marjoram. Also, try chopping or grinding fresh herbs if they are available, instead of using the dried or flaked form.

Another trick to flavoring comes in using ordinary fruits and vegetables as ingredients which serve surprisingly well as sweetners. Fruit juice is an obvious alternative to sugar. Not so obvious, though is the use of cooked carrots. They give a sweet flavor to soups and main courses which normally call for the addition of sugar, such as spaghetti sauce. If the carrots themselves should not be in the finished product, leave them whole and remove them after cooking but before serving the dish.

Other sweet vegetables can also be used, like sweet potatoes, yams and squash. Even sweet corn can sometimes serve the same sweetening purpose. Just omitting salt from the dish will automatically sweeten it and thereby simplify the job for you.

LET'S GET TO THE MEAT OF IT
======================================

We've already talked about the diet problems associated with meat. Meats are high in fat and calorie content, plus most meat is loaded with cholesterol. Of all foods to avoid, meat therefore, is at the top of the list. But remember, one of the objectives of this book is to offer a diet philosophy and recipes to live with indefinitely, not just during a brief weight loss program. Therefore, we will use meats in a way to satisfy the pallet while not hurting the diet.

Let's start by considering meat only as flavoring in a recipe rather than as the main ingredient of a meal. Think of meat as you would think of an herb or spice.

We'll talk about "meat" in three groups. First we have the red meats, including beef, pork and lamb. Next we have fowl, mainly chicken and turkey. Finally we have seafood as a group. In these recipes, the red meats are never called for. We even avoided using broth made from them. By way of a gen-eralization, red meat has about double the calorie content of fowl and about triple that of seafood.

Once you've tried these recipes without red meat and learned how much can be done using fowl and seafood, combined with other flavoring tricks, you will soon find you don't miss the red meat. In fact, it will probably become the least attractive item on a restaurant menu when you eat out.

Anytime you would be tempted to use hamburger, substitute chickenburger or turkeyburger instead. It satisfies the meat craving, imparts a good meat flavor and it contains less than half the calories and cholesterol. If that isn't enough good news, you will love knowing it only costs about half as much per pound as beef hamburger or pork sausage.

FABULOUS FIBER FOODS

The recipes in this book emphasize a reduction in foods which are high in fat, sugar and salt. They are replaced with fruit, grains and vegetables. As a result we not only minimize the harmful effects the former foods can cause to our bodies and reduce the calories we ingest, but just as importantly, we greatly increase the amount of fiber in our diet.

Food fiber comes from the structural parts of plants we eat, but which cannnot be dissolved by our digestive system. Once in our bodies the fiber tends to soak up liquids much as a sponge soaks up water. The result is to give bulk to human waste.

British physicians Hugh Trowell and Denis Burkitt did much of the early research which made people aware of the importance of fiber. Research is still ongoing, but indications are that the effects of fiber in the diet are mostly positive.

One of the first things you will probably notice when increasing the fiber in your diet is more of a "full" feeling as you eat. This of course, helps reduce your appetite and tends to reduce your calorie intake. People with a constipation problem may also notice more regularity due to the laxative effect which the fiber gives.

The positive medical and health aspects believed to be aided by more fiber in our diets include prevention of such problems as hemorrhoids, appendicitis, colon-rectal cancers, hiatus hernia, diverticulosis.

A diverticulosis disease is one in which the intestine walls become infected and is very common among Americans. Approximately 40% of of our population suffers from some form of this disease. At one time it was treated with low-fiber diets, but the current thinking is to emphasize high-fiber diets instead.

The recipes in this book remove most of the meats and processed food products which are high in calories and low in fiber. They are replaced with low-calorie, high-fiber foods. This is just another example of how you can lose weight and gain an overall improvement in your health.

EAT AND ENJOY !

LOVE YOUR VEGGIES

We've been talking at some length about the many health and weight-control advantages of vegetables over meats and sweets. The problem with changing our eating habits to include more vegetables comes in finding ways to make them more satisfying to our pallet. This brings us back to the primary objectives of this book, which are:

1. Lose weight
2. Keep it off
3. Eat healthier

This book is not for the "meat, potatoes and gravy" eater. It is for people who also want to achieve the objectives of this book. For many, this means a change in their thinking about food and what they like to eat. These people need to consider the harm they are doing to themselves by not eating right, then gain some appreciation for the good they can do for themselves when they change.

That's the first step in learning to LOVE YOUR VEGGIES.

Next we need to concentrate on making them more enjoyable and satisfying to eat. The trick is to do it without adding salt, oil or sugar and thereby negating the benefits of giving up meats and sweets. That's where the spices, herbs and use of natural flavorings come into play.

Some of the recipes in this book will surprise you when you read the combinations of foods or the flavorings to be used. Have faith, though, because each one has been taste-tasted by true food lovers and former meat-eaters, and judged to be delicious.

The psycological flavoring that comes from knowing you are eating healthier should greatly aid in the transition to a diet which is high in vegetables and other plant foods.

PASS THE POTATOES, PLEASE

=================================

Earlier we said these recipes are not for the "meat, potatoes and gravy" eater. We really should modify that statement and only eliminate the two of those old standbys that are bad for us, namely the meat and gravy. Then we should concentrate on the many ways we can eat and enjoy the one "good" food of those three, which is the potato.

Potatoes are probably the most maligned of all common foods. This is a result of those unhealthy high-fat, low-carbohydrate fad diets that were so popular in the '60s and '70s. The main thrust of those fads was to nearly eliminate carbohydrates or "starches". The common form of starch is white, the same color as a cooked potato. So it followed that potatoes must be bad for people on a weight-loss diet, right? Wrong!

The potato has one of the best balances of nutritional components of any food. Sweet potatoes and yams may come the closest to being "perfect" of all the foods we eat. They are made up primarily of slow-burning, low-fat, high-energy, complex carbohydrates. They also provide a good source of vitamins and minerals, especially potassium.

What we need to do, then, is prepare our friend the potato in ways that make us want to fill up on it and not feel cheated without the meat and the gravy. In this book the section of recipes on preparation of vegetables includes many ways to prepare potatoes which accomplish that very objective. Each recipe is simple, satisfying and naturally healthful.

Now it's time to reject the "old wive's tale" that potatoes are not the thing to eat when you want to lose weight. Old ideas, like old habits, die hard, but let's kill this one. So "pass the potatoes, please", and don't feel guilty about filling up on one of nature's most healthful food.

OODLES OF NOODLES

==================

Noodles, or pasta, in all shapes and sizes are recommended eating for a healthy weight loss diet. They are further recommended eating for life–long weight control. Pasta and rice dishes are prepared with the recipes in this book so extensively that they are each given an entire section.

Our earlier comments about the much maligned potato also apply to pasta and rice dishes. These are more of the slow–burning, low–fat, high–energy, complex carbohydrate foods we should all eat for a healthy life diet.

One of the beautiful things about pastas is that we have already developed a love for them. Think about spaghetti, linguine, fettucine or lasagna and you picture some delicious eating. Of course, anything that tastes that good must be bad for us, right? Yes and no. Prepared with salt, oil, eggs or sugar, the answer is YES. Follow the recipes in this book and the answer is NO.

Once you learn how to prepare delicious rice and pasta dishes by using herbs and spices instead of salt and oil for flavoring, you won't want to change. The reason is simple. You will be able to eat as much as you want (within reason) and not have to feel guilty about it. That's not a bad trade off. You give up some of the flavor you are used to, but you get to eat more of the food you love AND get a healthier diet out of the deal.

Don't forget another side benefit to eating those so–called "starchy" foods like potatoes, rice and pastas. Compared to meats and other oily foods, they are CHEAP. Everyone likes to save money, so add that ingredient called SAVINGS to the recipe and watch your enjoyment increase!

VALUE OF VITAMIN "X"

Losing weight and keeping it off starts with eating a diet of the right kinds of foods and eliminating the wrong kinds. But expecting to stay healthy through diet alone is like trying to clap with one hand. Once you've made the commitment to "eat right", take the next positive step toward better health and weight control. It's called exercise, or . . . VITAMIN "X".

Exercise is essential to building and keeping cardio–vascular systems healthy. Period. No argument.

So why don't more people exercise regularily? We hear many excuses, but they can all be combined under one of two possible categories. LAZY or IGNORANT. Too lazy to make the effort or ignorant of the reasons why exercise is so important to good health.

Much has been written about the positive effects of exercise on the human body. Likewise, the negative effects of not exercising are well chronicalled, so we won't repeat them in this book or discuss the statistics which have been developed by others.

Suffice to say that "X" is such a valuable ingredient in our "diet" that omitting it from our daily routine is like leaving the noodles out of spaghetti.

Everyone should use common sense or in some cases, get medical advice, then adjust their exercise level to their physical capabilities. People who can walk should walk. It's as simple as that.

A rapid walk sustained for 30 minutes or more works the large leg muscles, causing the heart to deliver more blood to them, so they work like pumps. The heart is a muscle, too, and this is the kind of exercise it needs to keep strong.

Other forms of exercise may be more beneficial, but often require better physical condition or more elaborate facilities. Take advantage of them if you are able, but if not, at least make a commitment to one of our simplest and most natural forms of exercise. Do the natural thing. Take a walk, and . . . take your VITAMIN " X" at the same time.

LET'S CALCULATE CALORIES

Calories do count, so don't let anyone tell you otherwise. The approximate calorie count in a serving is given with some of the recipes in this book as a guide and as you read them you will be pleasantly surprised by how low they are. Nevertheless, all natural foods have some calories, so if you want to eat more and still lose weight the secret is to burn off more calories.

Let's use some generalizations and approximations to simplify the process of adding and subtracting calories. Then we can set some goals for losing weight and keeping it off. For example, let's say:

1. There are 3,500 calories in a pound of fat.
2. Without exercise our normal bodily functions burn off ten times our weight in calories (a 150 pound person would burn off 1,500 calories).
3. Walking will burn off 100 calories per mile.

Now let's take a person who weighs 160 pounds, walks two miles twice a day and eats 1,500 calories. That person will burn off 500 calories more than he or she consumed that day. (160 pounds X 10 = 1,600; 2 miles X 2 times X 100 = 400; 1,600 + 400 = 2,000 calories burned off.)

500 calories is one–seventh of a 3,500 calorie pound of fat. So repeat this program for a week and you can see how the numbers work out to result in a the loss of a pound. Maybe one pound doesn't seem like much loss in a week, but imagine doing that for three months and you could see a 13–pound loss.

If you want to lose weight even faster, increase the amount of your daily exercise to burn up more calories, reduce the calories you eat, or do both. Once you have stabilized at your desired weight, adjust your diet and exercise level to maintain it. Just apply the formula to your personal weight, eating habits and exercise program.

Counting calories can be fun when you think about more than just how many you eat. Think, too, about the ones you are burning off. You will be even more encouraged to exercise and help control the calorie balance.

FALLING OFF THE WAGON

The basic philosophy behind these recipes is to make major REDUCTIONS in the amount of "bad" food we eat, rather than trying to ELMINATE it entirely. This is possible by using herbs, spices and unusual food combinations, in order to make the food appealing and flavorful.

One reason for this philosophy is the fact that it would be nearly impossible, and totally impractical, to do so. Another reason is that it would make it that much harder to stay on the diet. It is better in the long run to stay with a weight loss program which includes small amounts of "bad" ingredients than to become frustrated and give up entirely.

This same philosophy of making the diet easy to live with applies to those times when it isn't convenient to be on one, or for special occasions, when you just "fall off the wagon". Everyone falls off occasionally, so let's expect it and not be too upset with ourselves when it happens. The objective is to keep those occasions to a minimum and to jump right back on the wagon after you've fallen off.

If you have weight to lose, try to be a 100 percenter. That is DON'T fall off the wagon at all for the first four weeks. If you've made good progress toward your total weight loss goal, reward yourself by selecting one MEAL a week to eat whatever you want. After another two weeks if you are still progressing, allow yourself one DAY a week off the wagon.

Once you've achieved your desired weight you should be able to maintain it by eating according to the recipes in this book throughout the week, then relaxing the rules during the weekends. You will probably find, though, that sweet, oily and salty foods won't appeal to you so much anymore.

So . . . don't suffer from guilt pangs when you eat an occasional fast food meal. Just hop back on the wagon in time to catch the next meal.

Now its time to get started, and . . .

READY – SET – EAT !

STOCKING YOUR PANTRY

The following is a list of items you should have on hand in order to make cooking the low fat, low calorie way easier. There is less temptation to cook with oil, sugar and salt if they are not on hand, and if the substitutes you should use are conveniently available.

The BRAND NAMES included in the list may not be available in all parts of the country, but you should be able to find similar products by other names. Simply substitute those alternate brands instead, and you should have no problems with the recipes.

SEASONINGS AND FLAVORINGS

SALT SUBSTITUTE
      (Morton's, Nu–Salt, Schilling Saltless)

SOY SAUCE – light, low sodium
      (Yamasa, Chun King)

NO–SALT SEASONING MIX – shakers
      (Mrs. Dash, Parsley Patch, Lawry's,)

BROTH MIX PACKETS – low calorie, chicken or beef
      (Romanoff, MBT)

SALAD DRESSINGS – bottled, no–oil, low–calorie, all flavors
      (Pritikin, Tasti Diet, Estee, and Henri's are best. S & W, Weight
      Watchers, Kraft, Walden Farms are okay.)

SPRAY COATINGS – non–sticking
      (PAM, Cooking Ease)

VINEGARS, FLAVORED – white, apple cider, tarragon

LEMON JUICE – concentrate or fresh lemons

GARLIC – Whole or powdered

SPICES and HERBS – The following list includes all the herbs and spices used in recipes which follow. Experiment freely to find your favorite combinations.

Paprika	Bay Leaf
Chili Powder	Onion Powder
Celery Seed	Cinnamon
Dillweed	Nutmeg
Cayenne Pepper	Chives
Basil	Parsley
Marjoram	Coriander
Tarragon	Caraway Seeds
White Pepper	Thyme
Tumeric	Rosemary
Curry Powder	Poultry Seasoning
Oregano	Cumin

DAIRY & EGG PRODUCTS

BUTTER – imitation only
    (Butter Buds, Molly McButter, Best O' Butter)

EGG REPLACER – powdered or liquid
    (Second Nature Liquid, Ener–G Powder)

MILK – nonfat, powder (Milkman)

COTTAGE CHEESE – low fat

YOGURT – nonfat, plain

STARCHES

RICE – instant or long grain, brown or white

PASTA – eggless, vegetable or whole wheat

CORNSTARCH

POTATO FLOUR STARCH

OATS – rolled

CORNMEAL

FLATBREAD – Norwegian

BREAD – Sourdough

RICE CAKES – low salt

SWEETS

SUGAR SUBSTITUTES
    (Equal, Sprinkle Sweet, Sugar Twin, Weight Watchers)

SPREADABLE FRUIT – any flavor
    (Smuckers)

APPLE JUICE – unsweetened

SYRUP – maple flavored
    (Estee, Cary's)

JAMS, JELLIES, PRESERVES – low calorie
    (Nutradiet)

EXTRACTS – vanilla, almond, rum, banana

OTHER FLAVORINGS

PIMIENTO – chopped or strips

MUSTARD – all flavors and brands

HOT SAUCE – all flavors and brands

POULTRY and FISH

CHICKEN – fresh or frozen, skinned, all parts

CHICKEN – ground, fresh or frozen

CHICKEN or TURKEY – meat chunks, fresh or frozen

TUNA – canned, water-packed only

CRAB MEAT – imitation, fresh or frozen

CLAMS – pieces, canned, water-packed only

BREAD, CEREAL AND GRAIN

SNACK FOODS – Rye Crisps, Matzo, Lavosh, salt-free pretzels

BREAD – whole grain, low calorie

PITA BREAD – whole wheat

TORTILLAS – corn and flour

CEREAL – hot and cold
       (see RISE AND SHINE for recommended brands)

GRAIN – bulgur, kasha and pearl barley

VEGETABLE and FRUIT PRODUCTS

VEGETABLES – all types, fresh and frozen, low-salt if canned

VEGETABLE JUICE – all types, low-salt if canned

FRUIT – all types fresh, no sugar added if canned or frozen

FRUIT JUICE – all types, unsweetened

TOMATO PRODUCTS – canned whole, stewed, paste and puree

PICANTE SAUCE – use the Pace brand or similar

MISCELLANEOUS

CLUB SODA and MINERAL WATER – low sodium only

EGGS – use the whites only, 2 egg whites = 1 egg

MILK – evaporated, low fat or skimmed

BAKING POWDER and SODA

COFFEE and TEA – decaffeinated

BEVERAGE MIX – all flavors, sugar-free
    (Crystal Light)

SOFT DRINKS – all brands, sugar-free, caffeine-free

RISE AND SHINE – IT'S BREAKFAST TIME

===================================

There is less variety in the breakfast meals on this diet than for the other meals of the day. However, if you keep a wide choice of cereals and a good selection of breads on hand, this important meal does not have to be boring. Some recommended cereals available in most supermarkets, which are low in fat, sodium and sugar include:

COLD CEREALS	HOT CEREALS
Product 19	Yellow Cornmeal
Shredded Wheat	Rolled Oats, regular
Grape Nuts	Roman Meal
Special K	Cream of Wheat, regular
Whole Wheat Flakes	Wheatena
Bran Chex	Health Valley Cereals
Health Valley Cereals	
New Morning Cereals	

Although no serving quantities are given here for the cereals, remember to use reasonable amounts. Remember the objective is to control your weight while you eat a healthy diet. 1/2 cup of fruit per 1 cup of cereal is the suggested maximum amount.

For variety add one or more of the following to your breakfast cereal:

> 1 teaspoon raisins
> 1/2 teaspoon cinnamon
> half of a banana
> berries, any type

Use only NONFAT MILK.

Use only ARTIFICIAL SWEETENER.

FRUIT AND JUICE SELECTIONS

Tomato Juice, 6 oz.
Orange, 1/2
Apple, small
Grapefruit, 1/2 (spiced grapefruit, see DESSERTS)
Berries, any variety, 3/4 cup
Melon wedge, any variety, 1/6
Tangerine, small
Peach, small, fresh, sliced
Pear, small, fresh

BREAD SELECTIONS

To be eaten plain or toasted. Use spreadable fruit or diet jams and jellies for flavoring. DO NOT use butter or margarine.

Sourdough
Danish Pumpernickel
Lavosh
Norwegian Flatbread
Rye Krisps
Wheat Breads (Check ingredients on the label and only buy those that are low in fat, egg, sweetener and sodium content.)

OTHER DAIRY PRODUCTS

YOGURT – plain, low fat (This can be used for variety by mixing it with 1/2 cup of any appropriate fruit selection, above.)

COTTAGE CHEESE – low fat, drained in collander (Mix this with fruit also, for breakfast variety.)

RICE PUDDING CEREAL

Make good use of leftover rice and cook up some of this cereal on a cold winter morning. It satisfies your sweet tooth also.

> 1-1/2 cups cooked rice
> 1 cup low fat milk
> 2 egg whites, beaten with fork
> Sugar substitute equivalent to 2 t. sugar
> 2 T. raisins
> 1/4 t. cinnamon

Combine all ingredients in a medium saucepan and mix well. Cook mixture over medium heat, stirring, until it has thickened (about 5 minutes after the milk reaches a boil).

2-3 servings

HOT SLICED APPLES

This dish is especially nice on cold winter mornings in lieu of grapefruit or berries, and it only takes a little time.

> 1 apple, peeled, cored and cut into bite sizes
> 1 t. apple juice (unsweetened) or water
> 1/2 t. cinnamon

Mix all ingredients together in microwaveable dish. Cover with plastic wrap and microcook on HIGH for 2 minutes and 20 seconds.

If you don't use a microwave, place the ingredients in a covered pan over medium heat until tender.

Serve with a dollop of low fat, plain yogurt if desired.

EGG DISHES

Use a NO-CHOLESTEROL EGG SUBSTITUTE, according to directions on the carton. Scramble or make omelet in a Teflon pan sprayed with a non-stick coating.

When using real EGG WHITES, beat till frothy, then scramble in a Teflon pan sprayed with a non-stick coating.

For equivalent measure, 2 egg whites equals 1 whole egg.

To the scrambled mixture add any of the following:

> 2 T. chopped onion
> 2 T. chopped pepper, green, red or yellow
> 1 T. salsa
> no-salt herbal seasonings, to taste
> 2 T.   sprouts
> 1 T. low fat shredded cheese (maintenance diet)
> salt substitute
> ground black pepper
> paprika

MUSHROOM SCRAMBLED EGGS

> 1/2 cup chopped or sliced fresh mushrooms (or 1/2
>   cup canned, drained)
> 4 egg whites, lightly beaten (or egg substitute equivalent
>   to 2 eggs)
> Fresh parsley or chives, chopped

To a small Teflon skillet sprayed with non-stick coating, add 1 T. water. Fry mushrooms in pan for 1 minute, stirring. Add egg whites or egg substitute and scramble. Serve at once, sprinkled with parsley or chives.

Serves 2.

SCRAMBLED EGGS WITH TOMATO – Serves 2-3

2 t. light soy sauce
1/4 t. each parsley, basil and oregano
2 T. minced onion
1 garlic clove, minced
1 tomato, chopped, mashed and drained
Pepper to taste
8 egg whites (or egg substitute equivalent to 4 eggs)

In 12-inch Teflon skillet sprayed with non-stick coating, add light soy sauce. Over medium to high heat fry herbs, onion and garlic for 30 seconds, stirring. Add tomato and fry 2 minutes more, stirring. Add pepper. Mix well. Add egg whites or egg substitute and scramble. Serve at once.

The following are a few recipes you may want to cook on weekends or for a special breakfast because they take a little more time. Of course, they are delicious and satisfying any day of the week.

FRENCH TOAST

Slices of sourdough bread
Liquid egg substitute, or powdered egg replacer made into a liquid, or
    egg whites beaten till frothy
Cinnamon

Dip bread in the egg mixture to coat. Place in a Teflon griddle or skillet sprayed with non-stick coating and sprinkle with cinnamon. Brown one side. Flip over, sprinkle with cinnamon and brown the other side.

As a topping use:

Spreadable fruit
Fresh berries and mock sour cream (see SAUCES)
LITE syrup, diluted with a bit of apple juice (may
    be heated)
Hot Spiced Apples (allow them to cook a bit longer
    so they have the consistency of applesauce)

COTTAGE CHEESE PANCAKES

 1 cup low fat cottage cheese, drained
 1/4 cup low fat milk
 3/4 cup all-purpose flour
 4 egg whites, beaten with fork till frothy
 1-1/2 t. lemon juice
 1 cup fresh berries
 Mock Sour Cream (see SAUCES)

Combine cottage cheese, milk and flour. Add beaten egg whites to mixture. Add lemon juice and stir gently. Spoon batter onto non-stick griddle or skillet. Turn when the top starts to bubble and the bottoms are lightly browned.

Serve, topped with fruit and Mock Sour Cream or low-cal syrup.

POTATO PANCAKES

This recipe is also good as a lunch or dinner main course with a bowl of Borscht.

 2 pounds potatoes, peeled and grated
 1 onion, grated into potatoes
 2 egg whites, beaten with fork till frothy
 4 T. all-purpose flour
 1/4 t. ground black pepper
 1/4 t. salt substitute

Stir beaten egg whites into potato/onion mixture. Stir in flour, pepper and salt. Drop batter by spoonfuls onto Teflon fry pan or griddle sprayed with non-stick coating. Brown one side, flip and brown on the other side.

Serve with unsweetened applesauce and/or Mock Sour Cream, or make your applesauce as described in the recipe for FRENCH TOAST, above.

NOTES
======

SUPER SOUPS and SAUCY SAUCES

================================

HOT SOUPS AND STEWS

ANY DAY VEGETABLE SOUP

1 envelope chicken broth mix (Weight Watchers) dissolved in 1
cup hot water
Choose as many of the following vegetables as desired:

1 medium turnip, peeled and diced
2 stalks celery, sliced
1 onion, diced
1 carrot, scraped and diced
1 medium potato, peeled and diced
1/4 head cabbage, shredded
Half of a 10-ounce package of frozen chopped broccoli
Half of a 10-ounce package of frozen cauliflower
1 small zucchini or summer squash, sliced
Half of a 10-ounce package of frozen corn
Half of a 10-ounce package of frozen peas

1 16-ounce can tomatoes, broken up
2 T. tomato paste
1/4 t. oregano
1/4 t. marjoram
1/4 t. basil
1/4 t. salt substitute
1/4 t. ground black pepper

Cook turnip, potato, celery or carrot in a deep pot with the dissolved
broth mix. (Add water to cover if necessary.) Simmer covered till vegetables are partially tender. Add remainder of vegetable choices, canned
tomatoes, tomato paste, 1/2 cup water per vegetable added, and seasonings. Stir. Simmer covered slowly for 40 minutes. Add more seasonings
to taste.

NOTE: You can substitute one of the herb and spice shaker mixtures for
the seasonings listed. Seasoning is all a matter of taste. Don't be afraid
to go heavy on them to accomodate the lack of fats and protein in the
recipe.

NOTE: Depend a lot on soups, even in the summer. They taste good, they're filling, and a big batch will last for several days in the refrigerator. For future convenience, most soups can be frozen in smaller batches and thawed for use at a later time. With a green salad and some bread, soup can become the main course. All of the soups listed are quick and easy to make.

MINESTRONE

1-1/2 cups chopped onion
1 cup thinly sliced carrot
1 cup chopped celery
2 garlic cloves, minced
3 packets chicken broth mix dissolved in 4 cups hot water
1 16-ounce can tomatoes in juice, crushed

Seasonings:
2 T. chopped parsley
1 bay leaf
1 t. basil
1/4 t. rosemary
1/2 t. salt substitute
1/4 t. ground black pepper

1 cup elbow macaroni (eggless)
1 medium zucchini, cut into chunks
1 20-ounce can white beans, drained

Into large pot or Dutch oven pour 1/2 cup of the dissolved broth. Add onion, carrot, celery and garlic. Cook over medium heat for 8 minutes, stirring often. Add remainder of broth, tomatoes and juice, and seasonings. Bring to boil then reduce heat. Cover and simmer 40 minutes. Remove cover. Add macaroni and boil 3 minutes. Add zucchini and beans. Cover and cook for 5 to 7 more minutes.*

Makes 10 cups.

* Some eggless pasta cooks faster than regular macaroni. Check the package and adjust accordingly. You may need to add the pasta after the zucchini and beans have cooked for 3 minutes. Cook the entire mixture for 3 to 5 minutes or for the time indicated on the pasta package.

CREAM OF ANY VEGETABLE SOUP

Recipes for two white sauces are given in the SAUCE section. These may be used as the bases in soups as well as being used as sauces.

Other thickeners for soups are:

> Cornstarch mixed with an equal amount of water
> Pureed mushrooms
> Pureed cooked celery
> Pureed cooked onions
> Mashed boiled potatoes
> Pureed cooked squash
> Sourdough bread cubes soaked in water

Just a small amount of thickener is needed to give body to a thin soup. A wide variety of them is used in the following soups.

Although the following recipe uses carrot puree, you may substitute other vegetable purees as desired. Some possibilities are listed above. Other purees include broccoli, cauliflower, spinach, or any combination.

CREAM OF CARROT SOUP

> 1 medium onion, chopped
> 2 packages chicken broth mix dissolved in 2-1/2 cups hot water
> 1 pound carrots, peeled and sliced
> 2 cups potatoes, peeled and diced
> 1-1/2 cups nonfat milk
> Salt & pepper to taste

In a large Teflon saucepan sprayed with non-stick coating, saute the onion for 5 minutes. (Add drops of water if the onions begin to stick.)

Add the chicken broth, carrots and potatoes to the onions. Bring to a boil, then simmer till tender. Transfer to a blender in small batches and puree. Return to saucepan. Add the milk and seasonings. Reheat but do no boil. Serve carrot soup with a dash of nutmeg.

Makes 6 cups.
Calories per 1 cup serving: Approx. 85

The following recipe is a variation of the CREAM OF CARROT SOUP.
Use whichever sounds most appealing to you.

CARROT BISQUE – Serves 2

> 1/4 cup chopped onion
> 1 cup carrots, sliced
> 1 packet chicken broth mix
> 1–1/2 cups water
> 1 cup nonfat milk
> 1 t. Molly McButter or other butter substitute

In saucepan, dissolve broth mix in 1–1/2 cups water over medium heat.
Add onion and carrots then cook till tender. Add milk and butter substitute. Mix. Liquefy all ingredients in a blender. Return to heat and
sprinkle with celery salt. Serve hot.

Garnish with a dollop of Mock Sour Cream (see SAUCES) if desired.
This soup may also be served chilled.

QUICK AND CREAMY CAULIFLOWER SOUP

> 2 cups sliced cauliflower florets
> 1/2 cup sliced green onion
> 2 packets chicken broth mix dissolved in 2 cups hot water
> 1/4 t. thyme, crushed
> 1 cup nonfat milk
> 2 T. cornstarch

In large saucepan place cauliflower, 1/2 cup of the broth mixture, thyme
and a dash each of salt substitute and ground black pepper. Cover and
cook over medium heat till cauliflower is tender. Stir in the remaining
1–1/2 cups broth and 3/4 cup of milk. Heat through. Stir the remaining
1/4 cup of milk together with the cornstarch. Stir into cauliflower
mixture. Cook uncovered over medium–high heat, stirring constantly, till
mixture begins to thicken and bubble. Serve hot.

3 servings.
Calories per 1 cup serving: Approx. 80

BLENDER BROCCOLI SOUP – Makes 4 cups

    1-1/2 pounds broccoli, stemmed and chopped
    3 packets chicken broth mix, dissolved in 3 cups hot water
    2 stalks celery, shaved and chopped
    2 green onion, sliced
    1/4 t. salt substitute
    1/4 t. white pepper
    Dash of mixed herb shake

Combine all ingredients in large saucepan. Cook over medium heat, covered, about 8 minutes. Transfer to blender in small batches, puree till smooth. Return to pan and warm through. Serve hot.

SUMMER SQUASH SOUP – Serves 2.

    4 medium, unblemished summer squashes, cut into 1" slices
    2 packets chicken broth mix dissolved in 2 cups hot water
    Black pepper

Place squash in saucepan. Add broth and bring to a boil. Cover, lower heat and simmer till squash is just tender. Puree ingredients in blender or processor. Return to pot and reheat. Do NOT boil. Garnish with pepper.

ONION SOUP – Serves 4-6

    3 T. light soy sauce
    4 onions, chopped or thinly sliced (or chop 2 and slice 2)
    4 packets beef broth mix dissolved in 4 cups hot water

In large saucepan place the soy sauce, 1/2 cup of the sliced or chopped onions, and 2 T. of the broth mixture. Heat slowly till the onions start to burn, stirring occasionally. Stir and continue to evenly burn the onions till well browned. Add remaining onions and another 1/4 cup of the broth. Stir, cover and simmer 5 minutes. Uncover. Stir until liquid has evaporated and onions are browned. Add remaining broth and simmer 20 minutes.

You can float 1/4 slice of sourdough bread sprinkled with 1/2 t. of Parmesan cheese if you forgo bread or crackers with the meal or are in the maintenance stage of your diet.

TURKEY-VEGETABLE-BARLEY SOUP - 6 servings

This soup can be a meal in itself, or serve with green salad or cole slaw and some Norwegian flatbread.

    5 packets chicken broth mix dissolved in 9 cups of hot water
    2 cups chopped cooked turkey (frozen is okay)
    2 cups sliced mushrooms
    1 cup sliced carrots
    1 cup sliced onions
    1 cup sliced celery
    1 clove garlic, minced
    2 t. poultry seasonings
    1 cup barley
    2 cups nonfat or skim milk
    1/2 cup cornstarch or potato flour

Combine first 8 ingredients in large pot or Dutch oven. Cover and simmer 1 hour. Add barley and simmer covered, one more hour. Slowly stir 1/2 cup of the milk into flour or cornstarch till smooth. Add to soup. Stir till well blended. Add the rest of the milk and bring soup to a boil. Continue to cook until thickened.

SPICY SEAFOOD STEW - 6 servings (150 calories per serving)

    3 packets chicken broth mix dissolved in 4 cups hot water
    3 T. tomato paste
    2 t. ground cumin
    1-1/2 t. minced garlic
    1 pound red-skinned potatoes, scrubbed and cut into chunks
    2 ears of corn, husked, cut into 1-1/2" pieces
    12 ounces shredded imitation crabmeat (thawed if frozen)
    4 green onions, cut into 1" pieces
    1 T. fresh lime juice
    4-6 drops hot pepper sauce

Mix broth, tomato paste, cumin and garlic in large saucepan or Dutch oven. Cover and bring to a boil over high heat. Add potatoes and corn, cover and cook 8 minutes or till vegetables are almost tender. Add crabmeat and green onions. Cook 2 minutes or till crabmeat is heated through. Remove from heat. Stir in lime juice and hot pepper sauce. Serve hot.

LENTIL SOUP

With a green salad and some of the recommended crackers or bread, this too makes a good main course soup.

1/2 cup garbanzo or white beans, dried, soaked overnight or for several hours in enough water to cover. Drain and cover again with water and cook for 1-1/2 hours. When half done add the following:

3/4 cup chopped onion
3/4 cup chopped celery
3/4 cup diced carrots
3/4 cup lentils, dried and rinsed
1/4 cup long grain rice, brown preferred
1 16-ounce can tomatoes, blended
2 T. lemon juice
1 T. vinegar
1 t. basil
1/2 t. garlic powder
pepper to taste
salt substitute to taste
6 cups water or more as needed

Cook the remaining 45 minutes.

Makes 8 -10 servings

HOT AND SOUR SOUP – 4 servings

> 3 packets chicken broth mix dissolved in 3 cups hot water
> 1/4 cup sliced pitted ripe black olives
> 1/2 cup diced tofu
> 1/2 cup green onions, cut into 1" pieces
> 1 T. cornstarch
> 3/4 cup water
> 2 egg whites, beaten slightly
> 1 T. rice or white vinegar
> 1/8 t. cayenne pepper

Place in large saucepan over medium heat, broth, olives, tofu and green onions. In small cup, combine cornstarch and water till smooth. Gradually add it to the broth mixture. Heat to boiling, stirring constantly until slightly thickened. Remove from heat. Slowly pour beaten egg whites into soup while stirring gently in one direction. Stir in vinegar and pepper. Serve hot.

BARLEY VEGETABLE SOUP – 8–10 servings (150 calories per serving)

This is an especially hearty and healthy soup. It's excellent when served with toasted sourdough slices.

> 4 packets chicken broth mix dissolved in 6 cups of hot water
> 1–1/2 cups raw medium–grain barley
> 2 cups tomato juice
> 1 cup chopped carrots
> 1/2 cup chopped onion
> 1/2 cup chopped celery
> 1 t. minced garlic
> 1/2 t. pepper, basil and oregano
> 1 14–1/2–ounce can tomatoes, drained and broken up
> 3 cups mushrooms, thinly sliced

In large saucepot or Dutch oven, bring broth and barley to boil over high heat. Reduce heat to low and simmer 30 minutes. Stir in remaining ingredients EXCEPT tomatoes and mushrooms. Cover and simmer about 35 minutes, till carrots and barley are just tender, stirring occasionally. Add tomatoes and mushrooms and simmer about 15 minutes, till mushrooms are tender.

VEGETABLE CHOWDER

If you have some leftover chicken around, cut into small pieces and add to this chowder with the corn and pimiento. Double this recipe and it will give you a week's worth of low-cal but filling and delicious lunches. Just add a few Rye Krisps or Pita Toasts.

1 packet chicken broth mix
1-1/2 cups water
1 cup frozen cut broccoli
1 cup sliced fresh mushrooms
1/2 cup chopped onion
2 T. all-purpose flour
1/2 t. salt substitute
1/4 t. white pepper
1 13-1/2 ounce can evaporated low fat milk
1 8-ounce can whole kernel corn, drained
1 T. chopped pimiento

In small saucepan bring broth mix and water to boil. Add broccoli, reduce heat, cover and simmer for 3 minutes. Add mushrooms and onion and simmer 2 minutes longer. Do not drain. Set aside.

Mix flour with salt substitute and pepper to taste in small bowl. In another pan place milk. Add flour mixture and heat till bubbling over medium-high heat, stirring constantly. Cook and stir 1 minute longer. Stir in broccoli mixture and broth, corn and pimiento. Heat through.

Serves 6.

TOMATO-SEAFOOD STEW

        1/2 lb. fresh or frozen shrimp, thawed and halved lengthwise
        1 cup chopped onion
        2 cloves garlic, minced
        1 16-ounce can tomatoes, cut up
        1 cup Homemade Tomato Sauce (see SAUCES) or 1 8-ounce can
            low-sodium tomato sauce
        1 medium potato, peeled and chopped
        1 medium green pepper, seeded and chopped
        1 stalk celery, chopped
        1 medium carrot, shredded
        1 t. thyme
        1/4 t. pepper
        Several dashes hot pepper sauce
        2 10-ounce cans whole baby clams

In large saucepan cook onion, garlic and undrained tomatoes for 5 minutes or till onion is tender. Add tomato sauce, potato, green pepper, celery, carrot, thyme, pepper and hot pepper sauce. Bring to a boil. Reduce heat, cover and simmer 20-25 minutes or till vegetables are tender. Stir in shrimp and clams. Bring to boil again. Reduce heat, cover and simmer 1-2 minutes more or until shrimp turn pink. Serve.

COLD SOUPS*
----

*Some may also be served hot.

QUICK VICHYSSOISE – Serves 2-3

        1/4 cup chopped green onions
        1 16-ounce can whole potatoes, drained
        1 cup nonfat milk
        1/2 t. salt substitute

Cook green onions in a bit of water or microcook till tender. In blender, at low speed, blend potatoes, milk, salt and cooked onions. Serve hot or cold. Garnish with more chopped green onions or a dash of celery salt.

QUICK BORSCHT

      1 16–ounce jar red cabbage, undrained
      1 16–ounce can julienne beets, undrained
      1 packet beef broth mix dissolved in 1 cup hot water
      2 T. white wine vinegar
      Nonfat, plain yogurt, optional
      Dillweed, crushed, optional

Combine ingredients in a large bowl. Cover and chill till ready to serve. Garnish with a sprinkle of dillweed or dollop of Mock Sour Cream or yogurt, if desired.

This soup is also good served hot in the winter.

6 servings.

GAZPACHO – Serves 2 (70 calories per serving)

Great in the summer.

      2 medium tomatoes, peeled, cored and coarsely chopped
      1 small cucumber, seeded and chopped
      1/4 cup finely chopped green pepper
      2 T. fresh parsley, finely chopped
      1 6–ounce can (3/4 cup) hot–style vegetable juice cocktail
      1 T. lemon juice
      1 small clove garlic, minced
      1/4 t. tarragon, crushed
      1/4 t. basil, crushed

Combine all ingredients in a bowl. Cover and chill.

BLENDER GAZPACHO

This soup can be served right from the blender if all the ingredients have been chilled beforehand.

> 1-1/2 cups tomato juice
> 1-1/2 cups spicy tomato juice cocktail
> 1 large cucumber, peeled, seeded and cut in chunks
> 1 large green bell pepper, seeded and cut in chunks*
> 1 small onion, cut in chunks
> 2 T. lemon juice

Process all ingredients in blender (in batches if necessary) till vegetables are coarsely chopped. Serve immediately or transfer to a bowl and chill.

A food processor may be used instead of a blender. Be careful not to over-process.

Serves 4.
Calories per serving: Approximately 56

* You may use yellow bell pepper instead of, or in addition to, the green pepper.

NOTES

SAUCY SAUCES
===============

The following sauces are good to have on hand so you won't be tempted to reach for a can or jar of processed sauce, or for a package of dry mix. These sauces are salt free, fat free and sugar free, but taste so delicious you'll find it hard to tell they don't have those harmful ingredients.

HOMEMADE TOMATO SAUCE

> 2 large onions
> 2 garlic cloves, minced
> 8 cups peeled coarsely chopped tomatoes (or commercial brand peeled tomatoes equivalent to 8 cups. Make sure no sugar or salt has been added.)
> 1 T. oregano
> 1-1/2 t. salt substitute
> Artificial sweetener equal to 1 teaspoon sugar
> 1 t. basil leaves
> 1 t. rosemary
> 1/2 t. ground black pepper
> 2 cups water
> 1 12-ounce can tomato paste

In 4-quart saucepan or Dutch oven sprayed with non-stick coating, cook onions and garlic till tender. Add remaining ingredients. Heat to boiling, stirring occasionally. Simmer on low heat for 15 minutes.

May be stored in refrigerator for 1 week or in freezer for up to 3 months.

Makes 4-5 pints.

Calories per 1/2 cup serving: Approx. 65

NOTE: For a change, add some ground chicken (about 1/2 lb.) along with the onion and garlic, thus making a meat sauce.

For more variety, a can of drained, or a cup of fresh, sliced mushrooms, can be added along with the onion and garlic.

MOCK SOUR CREAM

Good as a garnish in soups, as a sour cream substitute on baked potatoes, or as a topping on french toast and pancakes. You will find it mentioned in many of these recipes. Be creative and add chopped fresh fruit for a more glamorous breakfast topping.

Use it also to mix into tuna for tuna salad or as a substitute for mayonnaise.

very good

1/4 cup nonfat milk
1 cup low fat cottage cheese, drained
2 T. lemon juice

Combine all in blender. Liquefy. Makes 1 cup.

NOTE: One of the following may be added for variety before blending:

1 t. minced fresh onion
1/2 t. curry powder
1 t. each onion flakes and parsley flakes and 1/4
t. paprika

SALSA

Not only is this a nice snack food with homemade tortilla chips, but it also makes a good addition to scrambled eggs, omelets and fajitas.

very good

1 16-ounce can whole tomatoes, undrained and chopped
3 sweet red peppers, seeded and coarsely chopped
1/2 medium onion, finely chopped
1 can 1 T. canned diced green chilies
2 fresh tomatoes, seeded and chopped
2 T. fresh lime juice
1/2 t 1/4 t. oregano
1/2 t 1/4 t. basil
12 sprigs fresh coriander, minced

Mix all ingredients. Serve with homemade tortilla chips. (See SNACKS)

WHITE SAUCE

Use this sauce as a base for soups or for creamed vegetables. It's also good as a base for cream sauces to go with fish and poultry dishes.

> 2 T. flour
> 2 T. nonfat milk powder
> 1 T. cornstarch
> 1 cup nonfat milk
> Dash of white pepper
> Dash of salt substitute or garlic powder (optional)

In saucepan combine flour, dry milk and cornstarch in 1/4 cup of the nonfat milk. When smooth, add the rest of the milk and mix well. Add seasonings and cook over medium heat, stirring constantly. As it begins to thicken, lower heat to very low and continue stirring and cooking till the sauce has thickened.

Makes 1–1/2 cups.

NOTE: When this sauce is being used as a base for cream soups, try adding dillweed, onion powder or other seasonings of your choice as it is cooking and has thickened a bit.

SIMPLER WHITE SAUCE

This sauce is more bland but works well as a base for soups.

> 2 t. potato flour
> 1/2 cup skim milk

Combine and cook till thickened, stirring constantly.

Makes 1/2 cup of a thin paste.

NOTE: Add seasonings as desired. Try a dash of salt substitute and a dash of white pepper as called for in the White Sauce recipe above. Onion powder, dillweed, garlic powder or a shake of mixed seasonings all work well.

"BUTTERY" WHITE SAUCE

This is a great buttery-tasting cream sauce for chicken or tuna. Add seasonings and some pimiento, then serve on a bed of rice or eggless pasta.

> 1 packet liquid butter substitute (Butter Buds)
> 3 T. flour
> 2 cups low fat or skim milk
> Salt and pepper to taste

Combine all ingredients in a saucepan. Heat, stirring constantly until thickened.

Makes about 2 cups.

TARTAR SAUCE

> 1 recipe Mock Sour Cream
> 1 t. minced onion
> 1/2 t. prepared mustard
> Dash of lemon juice
> Dash of garlic powder
> 1/2 small dill pickle, finely chopped (or 1/4 t. crushed dillweed)

Combine. Serve with fish. You may want to experiment with the seasonings, adjusting them to your tastes.

CATSUP

> 1/2 cup tomato paste
> 1 t. vinegar
> 1/2 t. apple juice concentrate
> 1/8 t. garlic powder
> 1/8 t. onion powder

Combine to desired consistency. Add more tomato paste to thicken. Adjust seasonings to taste.

GARLIC "BUTTER"

Brush this "butter" on slices of sourdough slices and toast. Sprinkle with paprika, oregano and basil for an Italian touch.

>   1 packet liquid butter substitute (Butter Buds)
>   1/2 cup hot water
>   1 large clove garlic, minced

Dissolve packet of butter substitute in hot water. Add the garlic and mix well.

Makes 1/2 cup "butter."

CLAM SAUCE

Great over pasta!

>   1 recipe Garlic "Butter"   (see above)
>   1 6-ounce can chopped clams, drained
>   1 T. chopped parsley

Combine all ingredients in saucepan. Heat to simmering. Serve hot.

SALAD SPECIALS

GREEN SALADS

Greens to use:
shredded cabbage
fresh spinach
red leaf, Boston or iceberg lettuce
escarole
chicory

Allow 1/2 cup per person.

Add any of the following, chopped or sliced for a total of 1/2 cup per person:

raw cauliflower
raw broccoli
green onion
cucumbers
green beans
asparagus tips, steamed
raw young peas
peppers, green, red, yellow
artichoke hearts, cooked

jicama
celery
carrots
tomatoes
parsley
sprouts
zucchini
mushrooms

USE BOTTLED DIET DRESSINGS. The no–oil brands are best. Be sure to check the labels for ingredients. Many varieties claim to be "diet" but contain sugar, oil and sodium. Use 1 T. dressing per person. Tossing the salad with the dressing keeps you from using too much at the table.

If you prefer you can make your own dressing combining vinegar or lemon juice with seasonings. DO NOT ADD OIL !

NOTE: Keep a baggie of fresh, trimmed, raw vegetables at your desk or handy in the refrigerator to nibble on when you get the "munchies". Eat as much of them as you like.

CHINESE COLE SLAW – Serves 8 (Calories per serving: 55 approx.)

    4 cups shredded Chinese cabbage
    1 8-1/4-ounce can crushed pineapple (in its own juice), drained
    1 8-ounce can sliced water chestnuts, drained
    1/4 cup sliced green onions
    1/4 cup reduced calorie mayonnaise
    1 T. prepared mustard
    1 t. grated ginger root

Combine the first 4 ingredients in a large bowl. Cover and chill. Meanwhile combine remaining ingredients for dressing. Spoon over cabbage mixture and toss to coat.

BASIL TOMATO SALAD

This salad is especially delicious in the summer when you can find (or grow) fresh basil.

    2 large tomatoes, peeled and sliced
    1 stalk celery, finely chopped
    2 green onions, finely sliced
    1/3 – 1/2 cup diet Italian no-oil salad dressing (enough to cover)
    2 T. basil (fresh if possible), chopped
    Lettuce

Marinate tomatoes in dressing, onion, celery, basil mixture for 2 – 3 hours. Drain off dressing and reserve. Serve sliced tomatoes on a lettuce bed with the reserved dressing alongside.

2 – 3 servings.

NOTE: To peel tomatoes, plunge them briefly into boiling water; peel will slip off.

STUFFED TOMATO SALAD

      2 medium tomatoes
      1/8 cup lemon juice
      1/4 t. pepper
      1 cucumber, peeled and finely diced
      1/2 cup Mock Sour Cream (see SAUCES)

Remove thin slice from the top of each tomato. Remove the seeds and some of the pulp. Mix lemon juice and pepper then pour into one of the tomatoes. Let it sit a minute and then pour mixture from it into the second tomato. Discard surplus lemon juice from second tomato. Invert tomatoes on rack and let them drain awhile. Fill the tomatoes with diced cucumber mixed with 1/4 cup of the Mock Sour Cream. Save the surplus to top the tomatoes. Arrange on lettuce leaves.

Serves 2.

CHICKEN SALAD WITH GRAPES

This can be served on a bed of lettuce or as a filler for whole wheat pita sandwiches. The chicken chunks can be found in the frozen food section or you may cook skinned chicken breasts and dice them after cooling.

      12 ounces (2 cups) cooked, diced chicken (white meat)
      1 cup chopped celery
      1/2 cup shredded carrot
      1/2 cup sprouts
      2 green onions, sliced in 1" segments
      1/2 cup grapes, cut in half
      1 t. lime juice

Toss all ingredients together. Serve with diet salad dressing of your choice.

Serves 4.
Calories per serving: Approx. 95 before dressing.

CHICKEN AND RICE SALAD

Serve this dish after you reach the maintenance stage of your diet – because of the mayonnaise.   Or use a mayonnaise substitute.*

       3 cups cooked brown rice
       2 cups (12 ounces) cooked chicken, cubed
       1/2 cup sliced celery
       2 T. sliced green onions
       1/4 cup diced red, yellow or green pepper
       1/4 cup no-oil Italian salad dressing
       1/4 cup light mayonnaise
       Lettuce

In bowl, combine rice, chicken and vegetables.   Mix together salad dressing and mayonnaise.   Add to chicken mixture and toss gently.   Chill.   Serve on lettuce bed.

4 – 5 servings.

* 1/4 cup low fat cottage cheese blended with 1/2 t. lemon juice and a dash of salt substitute.

QUICK TURKEY AND APPLE SALAD

       1 cup (6 ounces) frozen, thawed turkey chunks *
       3/4 cup chopped apple
       1/2 cup celery, diced
       1 T. raisins
       1/3 cup no-oil viniagrette salad dressing
       1 t. brown sugar
       Lettuce

In bowl combine turkey, apple, celery and raisins.   In cup, stir together salad dressing and brown sugar. Toss with turkey mixture. Serve on bed of lettuce.

2 servings.

* May use 1 5-ounce can chunky white turkey.

TUNA MACARONI SALAD – 6 servings (Approximately 230 calories per serving.)

8 ounces (2-1/2 cups) elbows or shells, cooked, rinsed, drained and cooled
1 13-ounce can solid white tuna, packed in water, drained, broken into bite-size pieces
1 7-ounce jar roasted red peppers, drained, cut into thin strips
1 small red onion, thinly sliced
1/2 cup diced celery
1/2 cup frozen peas, thawed
1/3 cup bottled no-oil Italian salad dressing
Lettuce

Mix all ingredients EXCEPT lettuce in large bowl. Toss gently. Serve on bed of lettuce.

SOY MARINATED CUCUMBER SALAD

1 cold cucumber, peeled, split lengthwise, thinly sliced
1 T. light soy sauce
2 t. cider vinegar
Pepper to taste

Mix all ingredients in a wide, shallow bowl and marinate for 5 minutes, tossing a few times. Serve salad in the marinade dish.

ASPARAGUS IN YOGURT

1/4 cup nonfat, plain yogurt
1 t. prepared mustard
1 t. Worcestershire Sauce
1 t. parsley, chopped
1 10-ounce package frozen asparagus spears, thawed
1/2 t. no-salt seasoning mix

Combine and mix yogurt, mustard and Worcestershire in medium bowl. In 10-inch Teflon skillet sprayed with non-stick coating, fry parsley over medium heat for a few seconds, stirring. Add asparagus and seasoning mix and fry 3 more minutes, stirring to cook evenly. Add asparagus to yogurt mixture and toss quickly but gently. Serve at once, hot.

CARIBBEAN SALAD

1 20-ounce can pineapple chunks in their own juice, drained
1 medium-size red onion, sliced
1 green pepper, seeded and cut into chunks
1/3 cup bottled no-oil or low-cal bottled Italian dressing
1/8 t. ground cumin
1 T. raisins, optional.
Lettuce leaves

Combine pineapple, onion and green pepper. Mix cumin and raisins into dressing; pour over salad and toss to coat. Spoon into lettuce-lined bowls.

4 servings.

NOTES
=======

VEGETABLE EDIBLES
====================

If you own one, use your microwave oven to cook vegetables. If you don't, steaming them is just as effective. Any vegetable can be cooked with these methods without using oil or salt, although salt substitute and other seasonings may be added after cooking.

STEAM vegetables in a covered pan, in water or broth mix to cover, until tender. The lists that follow include the timing for microcooking or steaming. They also suggest herbs and/or spices that can be added for taste and variety.

The vegetables should first be prepared for cooking: cleaned, trimmed and cut into pieces or slices, as appropriate.

For MICROCOOKING use microwaveable baking dishes – the amount of vegetable to be cooked determines the size. ALL DISHES should be covered with plastic wrap before heating unless stated otherwise. Become familiar with your microwave and adjust temperatures and cooking times to meet your personal requirements for the DONENESS of vegetables. Some people prefer their veggies crisper than others.

These recipes will provide for leftovers. Just reheat for the next meal. Be sure to add a few drops of water and cover the dish. Reheat to desired eating temperature, usually 1–1/2 to 2–1/2 minutes for microcooking and 5–10 minutes for steamed vegetables.

VEGETABLE/AMOUNT	MICROCOOKING METHOD and SEASONINGS
ASPARAGUS 1 lb. spears	Add 3 T. water. Cook 5 minutes, rearranging spears halfway through cooking. Let stand 5 minutes. SEASONINGS: Salt substitute, butter substitute, pepper, flaked tarragon.

VEGETABLE/AMOUNT	MICROCOOKING METHOD and SEASONINGS
BEANS, Green 1 lb.	Add 1/2 cup water. Cook 12–15 minutes, stirring every 5 minutes. SEASONINGS: Salt substitute, artificial butter, pepper, light soy sauce, garlic powder, pimiento, chopped cooked onion, sliced mushrooms.
BEETS 6 medium	Do not peel before cooking. Add 1-1/2 T. water. Leave whole. Cook 14–16 minutes, stirring after 6 minutes. SEASONINGS: Salt substitute, butter substitute, pepper, lemon juice, wine vinegar.
BROCCOLI 1 bunch, in pieces	DO NOT add water. Cook 8–10 minutes, rearranging spears after 4 minutes. Let stand 4 minutes, covered. SEASONINGS: Salt substitute, butter substitute, pepper, lemon juice, lite soy sauce, sesame seeds, chopped cooked onion.
CABBAGE 1 small head, cut into wedges	Sprinkle with 2 T. water. Cook 6–8 minutes, rotating after 3 minutes. Let stand 2–3 minutes. SEASONINGS: Salt substitute, butter substitute, pepper, wine vinegar, lite soy sauce, minced cooked onion, chives.
CARROTS 1 lb., sliced	Add 3 T. water. Cook 8–9 minutes, stirring after 4 minutes. Let stand 5 minutes, covered. SEASONINGS: Salt substitute, butter substitute, dillweed, ground ginger, lite soy sauce, sesame seeds, lemon juice, chopped parsley, chopped mint.

VEGETABLE/AMOUNT	MICROCOOKING METHOD and SEASONINGS
CAULIFLOWER 1 head florets 1 to 1-1/4 lbs.	Add 2 T. water. Cook 6–8 minutes, stirring after 4 minutes. Let stand 4 minutes. SEASONINGS: Salt substitute, butter substitute, pepper, dillweed, chopped chives, lite soy sauce.
CORN on the COB 2 ears	Wrap each ear in plastic. Place side by side on paper towel. Cook 3–4 minutes PER EAR. Rotate ears halfway through cooking. SEASONINGS: Salt substitute, butter substitute, pepper, mixed seasonings.
MUSHROOMS 1 lb., 1/4" slices	Add 2 T. water. Cover with waxed paper. Cook 4–6 minutes, stirring after 3 minutes. Let stand, covered, 2 minutes. SEASONINGS: Salt substitute, butter substitute, pepper, minced parsley, minced tarragon leaves.
ONIONS * 1 large sliced or chopped	Add 1 T. water. Cover with waxed paper. Cook 3-1/2 to 4 minutes. Let stand 2 minutes. SEASONINGS: Salt substitute, butter substitute, pepper, paprika, lite soy sauce, mixed seasonings.

* NOTE: Use onion as a flavoring for most foods, especially soups, rice dishes, casseroles and vegetable dishes. It's handy to keep at least a cup of chopped onions in the refrigerator at all times. Then you can quickly add them to recipes as needed.

TIP: A delicious, low calorie, no–fat side dish to almost any meal is onions, sliced and sauted in LIGHT Soy Sauce for 3 minutes. Add a bit of water, cover and simmer 6–8 minutes or till water is absorbed and onions are tender.

POTATOES – Since there are so many ways to cook potatoes, they will be covered later in the chapter.

VEGETABLE/AMOUNT	MICROCOOKING METHOD and SEASONINGS
SPINACH 1 lb.	DO NOT add water. Cook 5–7 minutes, stirring after 3 minutes. Let stand 2–3 minutes. SEASONINGS: Salt substitute, butter substitute, pepper, vinegar, lemon juice, chopped cooked onion.
SQUASH (acorn or butternut) 1 medium, cut in half length-wise.	Remove seeds. Place on flat plate, covered. Cook 10–12 minutes. Rotate after 5 minutes. Let stand 5 minutes, covered. SEASONINGS: Salt substitute, butter substitute, ground cinnamon, pepper, nutmeg.
SQUASH (summer or zucchini) 1 lb., sliced	Add 2 T. water. Cook 6–7 minutes, stirring after 3 minutes. Let stand 3 minutes, covered. SEASONINGS: Salt substitute, butter substitute, cooked minced onion, tomato sauce, Italian seasonings.
TURNIP (or rutabaga) 2–3 medium	Peel and cube. Add 3 T. water. Cook 7–9 minutes, stirring after 3 minutes. Let stand 2 minutes. SEASONINGS: Salt substitute, butter substitute, pepper, light soy sauce, chili powder, cumin, seasoning mix.

ARTICHOKES

These are good to serve to dieters because they take a long time to eat.

Cut off the stems and 1" of the tops; trim thorny tips. Wrap each one in plastic wrap. Microcook on High: 1 artichoke for 4 minutes; 2 for 6 minutes; 3 for 9 minutes or 4 for 12 minutes. Let stand in wrap 2 more minutes. Remove fuzzy choke with a spoon.

Serve with artificial liquid butter (Butter Buds) with a dash of lemon juice for flavor. Also, try blending some low fat cottage cheese with lemon juice seasoned to taste, as a dipping sauce.

STEAMING VEGETABLES

ARTICHOKES –	Do not steam. BOIL whole in water for 20 to 40 minutes.
ASPARAGUS –	Steam whole for 5–8 minutes, 5–7 minutes if cut up.
BEANS –	Steam whole 15–20 minutes, 10–15 minutes if cut up. (green or wax)
BEETS –	Do not steam. BOIL whole and unpeeled for 40 minutes to 3 hours, till tender.
BROCCOLI –	Steam stalks for 15–20 minutes, 10–15 minutes if cut up.
CABBAGE –	Steam quarters 25–35 minutes, 10–15 minutes if shredded.
CARROTS –	Steam whole 25–40 minutes, 15–35 minutes if cut up.
CAULIFLOWER –	Steam cut up 20–30 minutes.
CELERY –	Steam whole ribs 20–25 minutes, 15–20 minutes if cut up.
CORN –	Steam whole for 20–30 minutes. Or boil whole for 3–5 minutes, adding 1/2 t. sugar for each quart of water.

GREENS –	Steam leaves 15–20 minutes.
MUSHROOMS –	Steam whole 3–8 minutes.
ONIONS –	Steam small onions 25–40 minutes. Do not boil or steam large onions.
PEAS –	Steam large peas 15–20 minutes; small peas 5–7 minutes.
PEPPERS –	Steam halves for 15 minutes, 8–10 minutes if cut up.
POTATOES –	Steam cut up for 35–40 minutes.
POTATOES (new) –	Steam whole and unpeeled 25–35 minutes.
POTATOES (sweet) –	Do not steam. BOIL whole and unpeeled 25–30 minutes, 20–30 minutes if cut up.
SNOW PEAS –	Steam whole for 5–7 minutes.
SPINACH –	Steam whole leaves 15–20 minutes.
SQUASH (summer) –	Steam cut up 10–15 minutes.
SQUASH (winter) –	Steam cut up 25–35 minutes.
TOMATOES –	Do not boil or steam.
TURNIPS – (rutabagas)	Steam whole for 25–30 minutes, 15–20 if quartered.

ACORN SQUASH WITH APPLES

Cook one squash according to the microcook directions for Acorn Squash on Page 55.

Put the following mixture into a microwaveable dish:

> 1 cup apples, peeled and sliced
> 1 t. lemon juice
> 1/2 t. cinnamon
> dash of nutmeg

Cover and microcook on High for 2 minutes.

Fill the squash halves with the apple mixture and bake uncovered in a 350 degree oven for 15 minutes or microcook on High for 2 more minutes.

Serves 2.

EASY ACORN SQUASH

> 1 acorn squash (or other winter squash)
> 2 T. low-cal syrup
> 1 t. cinnamon
> Dash of butter substitute (shaker)

Preheat oven to 350 degrees.

Cut squash in half, wrap in plastic and microcook on High for 9 minutes. Remove plastic wrap, cover with foil and bake in conventional oven for 30 minutes. (If you have no microwave oven, bake covered with foil, in conventional oven for 1 hour.) Put some of the syrup, cinnamon and butter substitute mixture in each squash half. Place in oven, uncovered, for 5 more minutes. Serve hot.

MEXICAN TURNIPS

2 cups peeled and diced turnips
1/4 t. each coriander, cumin and chili powder
1/8 t. salt substitute
1/4 cup (1 ounce) shredded low fat cheddar cheese

Combine spices and salt. Set aside. Cook turnips, covered, in small amount of boiling water until tender (or Microcook 7-9 minutes in 3 T. water, stirring halfway through). Add spices. Toss to coat. Mash slightly. Sprinkle with cheese. Serve.

Makes 4 servings.
Calories per serving: Approx. 47

CARROT STUFFED SUMMER SQUASH

2 pounds carrots, cut into 1" pieces
1 T. water
1/2 t. diet orange marmalade
Salt substitute and white pepper
2 large summer squashes (or zucchinis)

Combine carrots and water, cover, and microcook on High for 10 minutes. Drain thoroughly. Puree in blender till smooth. Add marmalade, salt sub- stitute and white pepper, then blend. Set aside to cool.

Cut squashes in half and scoop out centers. Fill one half of each with the carrot puree. Put other half on as a lid. Transfer to baking dish. Cover lightly with waxed paper. Cook on medium (70% power) till heated through, about 2 minutes.

Serves 2.

SWEET AND SOUR VEGETABLES *

    1 medium onion, sliced (about 2 cups)
    2 medium carrots, sliced (about 1 cup)
    1 medium-sized green bell pepper, seeded and cut into chunks
    1/2 pound fresh green beans, trimmed and cut into 1" pieces
    1 large, tart green apple, cored and thickly sliced
    1 8-ounce can pineapple chunks in their own juice, drained
    1/4 cup white wine vinegar
    1/2 t. salt substitute

Combine onion and carrots in 2-quart microwaveable dish. Add 2 T. water, cover, cook on High till tender, about 4 minutes, stirring halfway through. Stir in bell pepper and beans. Cover and cook on High 3 minutes. Add apple, pineapple, vinegar and salt substitute, then stir well. Cover and cook on High till beans are crisp tender (or to your liking) about 4 minutes. Serve.

Makes 4 servings.

* TIP: If you add some imitation CRABMEAT, broken up, during the last 2 minutes of cooking you have a quick and easy oriental MAIN DISH.

SAUCY VEGETABLES WITH TOFU - 6 servings

    4 green onions, cut into 2" pieces
    2 medium carrots, thinly sliced
    1 small head cauliflower, cut into small florets
    1 small bunch broccoli, cut into small florets; slice stalks into
        1/4" pieces
    1 pound firm tofu, drained
    1 15 to 19-ounce can red kidney beans, drained
    1 8-ounce bottle low-cal creamy Italian dressing

Cut tofu lengthwise in half, then cut each half into 1/4" slices. In shallow 3-quart casserole, combine cauliflower, broccoli stalks and carrots with 1/4 cup water. In MICROWAVE, cover and microcook on High 7-9 minutes, stirring once. Stir in broccoli florets and onion. Cook, covered, on High, 3-5 minutes more. Drain. Stir in beans and dressing. Gently toss in tofu. Cook, covered, on High 5-7 minutes, till heated through.

APPLE-SWEET POTATO BAKE

This recipe takes some time only because the sweet potatoes need to be baked first for 50 minutes. You can do this a day ahead, or let the potatoes cook during your dinner time, fix the dish and have it all ready for the next day. It's worth the time and effort, is delicious and healthy.

> 1/2 lb. sweet potatoes (about 1 large)
> 3 Pippin or Granny Smith green apples, peeled, cored and sliced
> 1 T. apple juice
> 1 1/2 t. fresh lemon juice
> 1/2 t. salt substitute
> 1/2 t. cinnamon
> Dash nutmeg

Preheat oven to 375 degrees. Bake potatoes till tender, about 50 minutes. Peel and discard skin.

In microwaveable dish add apples and apple juice. Cover and cook till soft and mushy, about 5 minutes, stirring halfway through cooking. (Or cook in a skillet for 12 minutes, stirring occasionally.) Transfer apples to food processor. Add sweet potatoes, lemon juice, salt and cinnamon. Mix, using on/off turns, till smooth. Reheat if necessary. Serve hot with a dash of nutmeg.

Makes an excellent accompaniment with chicken or turkey.

Serves 2 to 3

POTATOES
==========

MICROCOOKING POTATOES

Pierce potatoes and place on paper towel. Arrange and cook on High as
follows:

1 potato	– in the center	– 4–5 minutes
2 potatoes	– side by side	– 6–8 minutes
3 potatoes	– triangle	– 8–10 minutes
4 potatoes	– in a spoke	– 10–12 minutes
5 potatoes	– in a spoke	– 12–15 minutes
6 potatoes	– in a spoke	– 15–20 minutes

Turn potatoes over halfway through cooking. Let stand 5–10 minutes covered
with foil or in a towel. Season with salt substitute, pepper, butter substitute,
Mock Sour Cream, chives, paprika, mixed herb shakes, garlic powder, or onion
powder.

POTATO TOPPERS

Whether you bake, boil or microcook your potatoes, here is a list of some low
calorie, low fat, low salt toppers you can add for variety and flavor. With
imagination you can make a great meal out of a potato.

– – A sprinkle of fresh dried herbs. There are many combinations sold in
shaker jars. Use them. Some that are especially good with potatoes are basil,
caraway seeds, oregano, celery seeds, dill, chives and thyme.

– – Low fat yogurt and chopped chives (fresh or dried) can take the place of
the more fattening sour cream.

– – Blend low fat cottage cheese till smooth and add 1 t. lemon juice. This is
another sour cream substitute. Add a dash of paprika.

– – A spoonful of Homemade Tomato Sauce (see SAUCES), a dash of basil,
oregano and garlic powder for a pizza potato.

– – Some chopped onion and sliced mushrooms sauted briefly in soy sauce.

– – A bit of water-packed tuna or salmon mashed with a bit of Mock Sour Cream and dried tarragon flakes.

– – Re-stuff baked potatoes after mashing the pulp with butternut squash and butter substitute or any of the toppers mentioned above.

NEW POTATO IDEA

Slit new potatoes across top to form a lid. Scrape out 1 T. of the potato. Sprinkle insides with a dash of black pepper, salt substitute, 1 t. butter substitute and one of the following:

chives	dill
tarragon	parsley
rosemary	

Replace lid.   Wrap potatoes in foil and bake at 425 degrees for 25 minutes.

TWICE-BAKED POTATOES – 4 servings *

2 large baking potatoes, about 1-1/2 lbs.
2/3 cups low fat cottage cheese
1/2 t. no-salt seasoning mix
Dash of salt substitute and pepper
2 T. sliced green onions
Paprika

Scrub potatoes, pierce and arrange 1" apart on paper towel.   Microcook on High 8-10 minutes until firm to the touch but easy to pierce with a fork. Wrap with foil and let stand 10 minutes.   Cut potato in half lengthwise. Scoop out potato, leaving a 1/4" thick shell.   Put pulp in a bowl.   Add cottage cheese and seasonings.   Beat till fluffy.   Stir in green onions. Spoon equal amounts into potato shells.   Sprinkle with paprika.   Microcook on High 2 minutes or till heated through.

*   If it's just the two of you, use one large potato and halve the rest of the ingredients.

POTATO AND TURNIP MASH - Serves 2

        1 large potato, peeled and cubed
        1 large turnip, peeled and cubed

Steam together in small amount of water till tender. Place in bowl while still hot. Add 1/2 t. salt substitute, 1/4 t. pepper and 1 t. butter sub-stitute. Mash all ingredients together.

For variety add chopped, cooked onion before mashing or a dash of any herb mix.

GREEN PEPPERS WITH SPROUTS

        2 green peppers, cut into strips
        1 T. light soy sauce
        1 cup bean sprouts
        1/4 cup tomato sauce, hot

In a 12-inch Teflon skillet sprayed with non-stick coating, fry peppers in soy sauce over medium heat, covered, for 3 minutes, stirring every 15 se-conds. Add bean sprouts and fry 1 minute, covered, stirring every 15 se-conds. Add tomato sauce and fry 30 seconds, stirring. Serve.

SPICED TOMATOES

        1 t. parsley, chopped
        1 t. basil (fresh if possible)
        1/2 t. oregano
        1/4 t. ground bay leaf
        1/16 t. ground cloves
        3 tomatoes, thickly sliced

In 12-inch Teflon pan sprayed with non-stick coating, cook spices over medium heat for a few seconds, stirring to mix. Add tomatoes and cook 4 more minutes, turning a few times. Serve hot.

CURRIED VEGETABLE BAKE

Can be made a day ahead and heated for 30 minutes at 350 degrees the next day. Although this is listed here in the Vegetable chapter, it is a main dish meal. It's full of protein and vitamins, so just add a tossed green salad and dinner is ready.

                3/4 cup dry lentils
                3/4 cup dry rice (not instant)
                Salt substitute
                3 small zucchini, sliced first lengthwise, then crosswise into 2"
                        pieces
                2 large sweet potatoes, peeled and cut into 1" chunks
                2 medium-sized red peppers, seeds removed, cut into 1" pieces
                1 small head cauliflower, cut into bite-size pieces
                1 small onion, minced
                2 t. curry powder
                1/2 t. cinnamon
                3 T. all-purpose flour
                2 packets chicken broth mix
                1/4 cup raisins

In 3-quart saucepan over high heat, bring 4 cups water to boiling. Add lentils, rice and 1 t. salt substitute. Heat to boiling. Reduce heat to low, cover and simmer 1 hour or until lentils and rice are tender and liquid is absorbed.

In 4-quart saucepan over high heat, bring sweet potatoes and enough water to cover, to boil. Reduce heat to low, cover and simmer 15 minutes or till potatoes are tender. Drain. In same saucepan over high heat, bring 2 cups water to boil. Add pepper, cauliflower and zucchini. Heat to boil. Reduce heat to low, cover and simmer 15 minutes, till vegetables are tender-crisp. Drain.

Meanwhile, in small non-stick skillet sprayed with a non-stick coating, cook onions, curry powder and cinnamon till onion is tender. (Add water to pan if it begins to stick) Stir in flour till well blended. Cook 1 minute. Gradually stir in 2 cups of water, then broth packets. Cook until mixture thickens slightly, stirring constantly to prevent sticking. Remove pan from heat and stir in raisins.

Continued on following page:

Preheat oven to 350 degrees. Spoon lentil mixture into shallow 3–quart casserole, pushing around the sides to form a border. Spoon vegetables inside of lentil mixture. Spoon curry sauce over vegetables. Cover tightly with foil and bake 30 minutes or till all vegetables are tender.

6 servings.
Calories per serving: Approx. 385

HERBED BAKED TOMATOES

This is an easy side dish for any meal, and takes the place of a salad or vegetable.

> 4 medium tomatoes – ends cut off and some pulp scooped out and reserved.

> Mix together:
>> sugar substitute equivalent to 1/2 t. sugar
>> 1/4 t. onion powder
>> 1/3 t. basil
>> 1/4 t. oregano
>> 1/8 t. black pepper
>> 1/2 cup Matzo crumbs (grind Matzo crackers in food processor)
>> Dash of butter substitute
>> Dash of parsley

Mix seasonings with tomato pulp. Stuff back into tomatoes. Top with Matzo crumbs. Sprinkle on butter substitute and crushed parsley leaves. Bake at 350 degrees for 20–30 minutes.

Makes 4 servings.

Calories per serving: Approx. 40

VEGETABLE ENCHILADA - 4 servings

        1 T. Light soy sauce
        4 small zucchini, cut into 2" matchsticks (about 4 cups)
        2 cups chopped green peppers
        1 cup chopped onion
        2 t. minced garlic
        24 ounces (3 cups) mild salsa (be sure check labels for
                                              oils or sugars)
        1-2 T. chili powder
        4 t. cumin
        8 corn or flour tortillas

Preheat oven to 350 degrees. In Teflon skillet sprayed with non-stick coating, add soy sauce and saute zucchini, peppers, onion and garlic till tender, about 5 minutes. Stir in 1/2 cup of the salsa, chili powder and cumin. Mix well and set aside.

Spray 9x13x2" baking dish with non-stick coating. Pour 1/2 cup of salsa in bottom of pan. Pour the rest of the salsa in a bowl. Dip each tortilla in the salsa. Spoon 1/2 cup of the reserved vegetables into the center of the tortilla. Roll up and place in pan, seam side down. Pour any remaining salsa over the rolls. Bake covered, until heated through, about 10-15 minutes.

Makes 4 servings.

NOTES
======

THE MAIN ATTRACTION
========================

PASTA DISHES
————————

There are many varieties of eggless pasta on the market. Some are sold in grocery stores; many are sold in stores specializing in "health foods." Use whole wheat, spinach or other vegetable pasta. It is a myth that pastas are fattening. What's fattening is the butter, oils and sauces we put on them.

BE CAREFUL when cooking eggless pastas. Many times they only need to be cooked for a short time and will break apart if they cook too long. Follow package directions closely.

SAUCY SPAGHETTI *

8-ounce package eggless spaghetti or linguine cooked according to package directions.
1 cup Homemade Tomato Sauce (see SAUCES)
1/2 lb. ground chicken, crumbled and cooked over medium heat (no oil added), drain any fat that cooks out
1/2 cup chopped onion, added to ground chicken while cooking

On plate place a portion of noodles, top with 1/2 cup tomato sauce and half the chicken mixture.

Serves 2.

* Spaghetti is just a type of pasta. Feel free to substitute vermicelli, linguine or other shape of your choice for the spaghetti noodle.

LEFTOVER SPAGHETTI

It's nice to have leftovers in the refrigerator. There's nothing better than coming home from work and finding dinner preparation is already half done you.

> 2 cups leftover cooked spaghetti or linguine
> 3 T. light soy sauce
> 3 green onions, sliced
> 1/2 cup sliced mushrooms (canned or fresh)

Saute onions and mushrooms in soy sauce till tender. Add spaghetti and toss till heated through.

OPTIONS: Add 1/2 cup crumbled imitation crab or cooked, chopped chicken when sauteing onion and mushrooms.

CHINESE SPAGHETTI

> 1 8-ounce package spaghetti, cooked according to package, drained
> 1/2 lb. mushrooms, sliced (or 1 8-ounce can, drained)
> 3 green onions, cut into 2" pieces
> 1 medium carrot, shredded
> 1 cup small shrimp, cooked
> 1/4 cup light soy sauce
> 1/2 t. sugar
> 1/4 t. crushed red pepper

In 12" skillet sprayed with non-stick coating, over medium heat, cook mush-rooms, onions and carrot till tender-crisp, stirring frequently. Add shrimp and cook 1 minute. Add soy sauce, sugar and pepper to skillet and toss with vegetables till heated through. Spoon mixture into saucepan with spaghetti. Toss to cover. Serve warm or refrigerate to serve chilled later.

3-4 servings.

PASTA WITH VEGETABLES AND CLAMS

The garlic is what gives this dish the flavor, so you don't miss the cheese.

This main dish makes a delicious and easy meal with a tossed salad with no-oil dressing and a slice of sourdough bread rubbed with a garlic clove and toasted.

1 green bell pepper, chopped
1 small red onion, chopped
1 lb. mushrooms, sliced
4 cloves garlic, minced
1-1/2 t. garlic powder
1/4 cup liquid butter substitute (Butter Buds)
1 10-ounce can chopped clams, drained (reserve liquid)
Salt substitute and pepper
1/2 lb. fusili pasta (or other comparable shape), freshly cooked
1/2 cup low fat shredded mozzarella (optional)

Combine first 5 ingredients in large glass bowl. Add the butter substitute and cover bowl with plastic wrap. Microcook on High for 2 minutes. Stir and cover again. Cook 2 more minutes. Mix in reserved clam juice. Stir, cover and cook on High 3 more minutes. Stir in chopped clams. Season with salt substitute and pepper to taste. Cover and cook on High 1 minute. Toss with cooked pasta. Serve immediately.

OPTION: If you are in the maintenance stage of your diet, add the shredded cheese and toss.

4 servings.

SPINACH FETTUCINE WITH SHRIMP AND VEGETABLES

      2 ounces dry spinach fettucine, prepared according to package, drained, keep warm
      1 t. cornstarch
      1/2 cup unsweetened orange juice
      4 large shrimp, peeled, deveined and sliced in half lengthwise
      1/2 cup snow peas
      1/2 cup chopped tomatoes
      1 carrot, shredded
      1/4 cup fresh mushrooms, thinly sliced

Blend cornstarch and orange juice together till smooth; set aside. In Teflon skillet, sprayed with non-stick coating over high heat, saute shrimp, snow peas and tomato just until shrimp curl and become opaque (about 2 minutes). Stir in orange sauce; cook till sauce thickens, about 1 minute. When pasta is just about done, toss in the shredded carrots; cook 1 more minute and drain. Toss with shrimp/sauce mixture, add mushrooms and season with fresh ground pepper.

2 servings.
Calories per serving: Approx. 220

SPAGHETTI VINAIGRETTE – 4–6 servings (125 calories per serving)

      1 8-ounce package spaghetti, prepared according to directions
      1 9-ounce package frozen artichoke hearts, prepared as label directs
      6 ounces radishes, sliced
      3 celery stalks, sliced
      1/3 cup chopped parsley
      3 T. cider vinegar
      1 packet sugar substitute (2 t.)
      1 t. salt substitute
      1/4 t. cracked pepper
      1 T. sliced ripe olives

In large saucepan with a steam basket, steam celery and radishes until tender-crisp. Do not overcook. Add artichoke hearts and celery/radish mixture to spaghetti. Toss gently. Add remaining ingredients and toss again. Serve spaghetti warm or refrigerate and serve later, chilled.

PASTA WITH TUNA AND TOMATOES – Serves 4

12 ounces thin spaghetti (eggless)
1 can water–packed tuna, drained
2 t. capers, drained
2 t. minced garlic
1 t. dried basil leaves
1 28–ounce can tomatoes, broken up, not drained

Cook spaghetti according to package directions, till tender but still firm. Drain and rinse with warm water. Transfer to serving bowl and keep warm. Meantime in Teflon skillet sprayed with non–stick coating, add tuna, capers, garlic and basil. Cook, stirring gently till well blended and thoroughly heated, about 1 minute. Add tomatoes and bring to boil. Cook 4–5 minutes longer till a smooth sauce is formed. Serve over spaghetti.

GREEN ON GREEN PASTA – Serves 4

12 ounces spinach linguine *
2 cups fresh broccoli florets
1 cup fresh asparagus, cut into 1" pieces
2 cups sliced zucchini
1/2 cup fresh snow peas
1/2 cup frozen, thawed green peas

Half of the White Sauce recipe (see Page 42).

Bring a large pot of water to boil. Add the linguine and cook 5 minutes less than time on the package.** While water is boiling add the broccoli and asparagus. Cook 2 minutes more. Gradually add the zucchini, snow peas and green peas then cook 3 more minutes.

Drain pasta and vegetables well; pour into serving bowl. Add White Sauce mixture and toss to coat. Serve immediately.

* Use regular linguine if you can't find the spinach kind.

** Make sure that the time called for cooking the linguine is more than 5 minutes. Many eggless pastas only need to be cooked for 3 minutes. In that case, add pasta 3 minutes before cooking is done.

PASTA WITH PEAS AND SCALLIONS

        3/8 pound eggless linguine, spaghetti, fettucine or other pasta of choice, cooked according to package
        1/4 t. parsley
        1/8 t. basil
        1/8 t. oregano
        1/2 of a 10-ounce package frozen peas, thawed
        2 scallions, cut into strips
        1/2 packet chicken broth mix dissolved in 1/4 cup hot water
        2 T. tomato paste
        Salt substitute and pepper to taste

While pasta cooks, in small Teflon pan sprayed with non-stick coating, cook herbs, peas and scallions for 3 minutes over medium heat. Add spoonfuls of the broth mixture if vegetables begin to stick. Blend tomato paste into broth mix and add to pan after 3 minutes. Add salt substitute and pepper then heat through, mixing well. Toss with cooked pasta and serve hot.

Serves 2.

PASTA WITH TUNA SAUCE

        3/8 pound eggless vermicelli, spaghetti, linguine or pasta of your choice, cooked according to package directions
        1 garlic clove, minced
        1/2 cup sliced mushrooms
        1 7-ounce can water-packed tuna, drained and flaked
        2 T. tomato puree
        No-salt seasoning mix to taste

While pasta cooks, fry garlic in a small Teflon pan sprayed with non-stick coating for a few seconds over high heat, stirring constantly. Lower heat to medium and add mushrooms. Fry 2 more minutes, stirring. Add tuna and fry 1 minute more, stirring. Mix in tomato puree and seasoning. Heat through. Toss with cooked pasta and serve hot.

Serves 2.

NOTES
=======

RICE DISHES

It is wise to keep a big bowl of rice in the refrigerator. It will last a week or more, but you will probably use it up in a few days. Brown rice is the best, but use the "instant" or "quick" rices to minimize preparation and cooking time.

ORIENTAL RICE AND VEGETABLES

This makes a good side dish for broiled fish or chicken.

> 3 T. light soy sauce
> 1 small onion, thinly sliced
> 1 stalk celery, chopped
> 1/2 cup sliced mushrooms
> 1-1/2 cups rice, cooked and drained

In Teflon pan sprayed with non-stick coating, add 2 T. of the soy sauce. Over medium heat, saute the onion for 1 minute. Add the celery and saute for 2 minutes. Add 1/4 cup water and cook for 5 more minutes on lower heat. Add the mushrooms and simmer 3 more minutes. Add the rest of the soy sauce and stir. Add the rice and stir till heated through. Serve hot.

Serves 2 with leftovers. (Heat leftovers for a quick lunch.)

NOTE: To make this a main dish add 6-8 ounces imitation crabmeat to the mixture when you add the mushrooms. Add 1/2 cup more rice.

BE CREATIVE: You can substitute or add any of the following ingredients either along with, or instead of, the ones above.

> pea pods
> frozen peas, thawed
> frozen or fresh corn
> carrots, scraped and minced (add at same time as celery)
> leftover broiled chicken, cut into bite-size pieces
> sprouts
> sliced zucchini (add at same time as celery)

RICE IDEAS

The following are based on 2-cup size rice recipes.

Raisin Rice – – Add 2 T. raisins to the water before bringing to a boil. Sprinkle with nutmeg, cinnamon or cardamon after cooked.

Minted Rice – – Add 2 T. chopped mint leaves when you add the rice. For more sweetness, add sugar substitute equivalent to 1/2 t. sugar.

Parsley Rice – – Add 2 T. chopped fresh parsley when you add the rice.

Chive Rice – – Add 2 T. finely chopped chives to rice just before serving and mix gently.

Apple Rice – – Add 1-1/2 cups finely diced unpeeled red apples to water before bringing to a boil. Add rice and cook according to directions.

Celery Rice – – Saute 1/2 cup chopped celery in 1 t. soy sauce and 1 T. water until tender. Add to water before bringing to a boil. Add rice and cook according to directions.

RICE WITH CARROTS

1 large carrot, scraped and thinly sliced
1 packet low-cal chicken broth mix
Dash cinnamon
Dash allspice
1 cup rice, cooked and drained

Put carrot in saucepan with enough water to cover, add the packet of broth mix and cook. Add spices and bring to a boil. Simmer till carrots are tender. Drain off liquid, add the rice and heat through.

Serves 2.

CHILI RICE AND BEANS

    3 cups cooked rice, still hot
    2 cups cooked beans (pinto, red or kidney)
    2 cups Homemade Tomato Sauce (see SAUCES)
    1 large onion, chopped
    1 medium green pepper, chopped
    1/2 t. chili powder

Combine all ingredients except rice. Heat through and pour over bed of rice.

6 servings.

BULGUR PILAF

    1 cup bulgur (cracked wheat)
    1 T. light soy sauce
    2 packets chicken broth mix dissolved in 2 cups hot water
    2 medium carrots, shredded
    1 stalk celery, finely chopped
    1 small onion, finely chopped
    2 T. chopped fresh parsley
    1/2 t. salt substitute

Preheat oven to 350 degrees.

In large ovenproof skillet sprayed with non-stick coating, saute bulgur in soy sauce for 5 minutes till lightly browned, stirring occasionally. Stir in broth, vegetables and salt. Bring to a boil. Cover and bake in oven 25 minutes or till broth is absorbed, stirring occasionally.

4 servings.

RICE PILAF WITH YOGURT – Serves 2

This is a good accompaniment to chicken kabobs. (see POULTRY)

> 1 cup rice
> 1 small onion, chopped
> 2 packets chicken broth mix dissolved in 2 cups hot water
> 1/2 – 1 cup plain, low fat yogurt
> Paprika

Cook onions in 1/4 cup of the broth till tender (or use microwave – see VEGETABLES). In saucepan combine rice, onions and remainder of broth. Cover tightly and cook over low heat till rice absorbs the liquid (about 20 minutes). Serve hot, covered with yogurt and a sprinkling of paprika.

BAKED BARLEY PILAF – 6-8 servings

> 3 T. light soy sauce
> 1-1/2 cups mushrooms, sliced
> 1 onion, chopped
> 3/4 cup scallions, chopped, green and white sections
> 2 carrots, halved lengthwise and thickly diced
> 1-1/2 cups barley
> 1-1/2 cups leftover chicken or turkey, optional
> 2 packets chicken broth mix dissolved in 2-1/4 cups hot water
> Salt substitute and pepper to taste

Preheat oven to 350 degrees.

In a skillet sprayed with non-stick coating, add the soy sauce. Saute mushrooms till almost tender. Set aside. Saute onion and scallions and carrots in same pan till onions soften, about 8 minutes. Add a bit of broth as needed if vegetables begin to stick. Add barley and saute, stirring for 6 minutes, till browned.

Pour barley mixture into 2-1/2 quart casserole. Stir in mushrooms and their liquid (if any), meat if desired, the remaining broth, 1 cup water then salt substitute and pepper to taste. Stir. Cover and bake till barley is tender, about 45 minutes. Check occasionally. If mixture dries out before cooking time is up, add more water. Add more salt substitute if desired.

QUICK RICE WITH VEGETABLES

        1 packet chicken broth mix dissolved in 3/4 cup hot water
        3/4 cup quick–cooking rice
        1/2 10–ounce package frozen, chopped mixed vegetables, thawed
        Butter substitute

Cook rice on stove or in microwave oven according to package directions, using the broth mix as the liquid. Add vegetables to cooked rice and cook till heated through. Sprinkle with butter substitute and blend well. Serve hot.

2 servings.

TOMATO RICE

This is a great accompaniment for broiled fish.

        3/4 cup tomato juice
        1/4 t. salt substitute
        3/4 cup quick–cooking rice
        1/4 t. parsley
        1/8 t. oregano
        1/8 t. basil
        1/4 cup chopped onion
        2 garlic cloves, minced
        1 cup coarsely chopped tomatoes and their juices

Mix salt substitute into tomato juice in a pan. Stir in rice, cover and cook according to package directions. Meanwhile, in 10–inch Teflon skillet sprayed with non–stick coating, fry herbs, onion and garlic over medium to high heat for 30 seconds, stirring. Add tomatoes and their juices and fry 2 more minutes, stirring. When rice is done, toss in pan with tomato mixture. Serve hot.

2 servings.

RICE WITH RED AND GREEN PEPPERS

A very colorful dish; delicious too!

>   1 packet chicken broth mix dissolved in 1 cup hot water
>   3/4 cup quick cooking rice
>   1/4 t. parsley
>   1 green pepper, seeded and cut into bite-size pieces
>   1 red pepper, seeded and cut into bite-size pieces

Cook rice according to package directions, using 3/4 cup of the broth as the liquid. Meanwhile, in a 10-inch skillet, cook parsley and peppers in the remaining 1/4 cup of the broth for 3-4 minutes. When rice is done, put into pan with peppers and toss. Serve hot.

Serves 2.

CRUNCHY BROWN RICE

This is an especially nutritious rice dish. Serve it with broiled chicken or add cooked shrimp to the mixture near the end of the cooking time and heat through for a main dish meal.

>   2 packets chicken broth mix dissolved in 2-1/2 cups hot water
>   3-4 green onions, sliced (include the green part)
>   1 cup brown rice
>   1/4 cup fresh or frozen (thawed) corn
>   1/4 cup nonfat dry milk powder
>   1 cup chopped tomato
>   1/4 cup fresh basil (or 2 t. dried)
>   1 small can water chestnuts, drained and chopped

Combine broth and onion in large pan and bring to a boil. Stir in the rice. Reduce heat, cover and simmer for 30 minutes. Add corn, milk powder, tomato, basil and water chestnuts. Simmer for about 10 minutes, or until rice is tender.

Serves 4.

NOTES
======

POULTRY

It's handy to have some cooked chicken on hand for a quick meal. With a pasta or rice dish and a vegetable or salad it makes a quick, nutritious meal. It's a great food to pack in a lunch or take on a picnic. Make sure you skin the chicken before cooking, and pour off any fat that comes out after it cooks.

BROILED CHICKEN (or GRILLED) – Serves 2, with leftovers

> 2-1/2 to 3 lb. frying chicken, cut up and skinned
> No-oil salad dressing – Italian, Creamy Italian, French or Russian

Coat chicken pieces with dressing of your choice. Cover and refrigerate at least 1 hour. Broil on rack or in pan sprayed with non-stick coating and broil 6" from heat 20 minutes on each side, till done.

Or grill on barbecue same amount of time.

BAKED CHICKEN * – Serves 2, with leftovers

> 2-1/2 to 3 lbs. chicken, cut up and skinned
> 1/4 cup flour
> 1/4 cup cornmeal
> 1 t. paprika
> 1 t. basil leaves
> 1/2 t. salt substitute
> 1/4 t. pepper

Preheat oven to 350 degrees. Toss all ingredients, except chicken, together in a small paper bag. Moisten chicken with water or nonfat milk. Place 1 piece at a time in paper bag and shake. Put coated pieces in a baking dish sprayed with non-stick coating. Bake for 50 minutes, till tender and cooked through.

* Another good coating for baked chicken is rolled oats (1 cup), 2 T. fresh parsley (or 1 T. dry parsley flakes) and 1/8 t. garlic powder processed in a blender or food processor to a cornmeal consistency.

CHICKEN CACCIATORA – 6–8 servings

This recipe makes up a big casserole. It will serve 2 people 3 times. Just store in an ovenproof dish and reheat at 350 degrees till heated through.

2 cloves garlic, minced
1 medium chicken, cut up and skinned
3 cups Homemade Tomato Sauce (see SAUCES)
1/2 medium green pepper, cut into strips
1/2 medium onion, chopped
1/4 t. oregano
1 bay leaf
1–1/4 t. basil
Salt substitute and pepper to taste
1 package (16 ounces) spaghetti, cooked according to directions, drained

In a large Dutch oven sprayed with non–stick coating, saute garlic. Brown chicken on all sides. Toss about occasionally to prevent sticking. Drain any fat that accumulates. Add Sauce, pepper, onion and seasonings. Simmer, covered, 40 minutes. Stir occasionally. Serve over cooked pasta.

LIME CHICKEN – Serves 2

2 boneless and skinless breasts, 1/2 lb. each (Frozen breasts may be purchased and thawed)
Juice of 2 limes
1 T. bottled lime juice
2 cloves garlic, minced
1 T. fresh cilantro, chopped (or 1 T., dried & crushed)
1/4 t. salt substitute
1/4 t. pepper

Trim all fat from breasts, cut out middle tendon. Pound between waxed paper till flattened slightly. Combine lime juice, 2 T. water, 1/2 T. cilantro, salt substitute and pepper. Pour over chicken and marinate at least 1 hour. Broil 2 minutes on each side, or till done. Serve with remainder of cilantro sprinkled over breasts.

CHICKEN AND RICE MEAL IN A SKILLET

2 lbs. meaty chicken pieces, skinned
3 cups fresh mushrooms, sliced
4 medium carrots, peeled and sliced 1/2" thick
1/2 cup chopped onion
3/4 cup long grain rice
1 packet chicken broth mix
1 t. poultry seasoning

Spray a 12" skillet with non-stick coating. Brown chicken pieces on all sides over medium heat about 15 minutes. Toss about to keep from sticking. Remove chicken and drain off any accumulated fat. To same skillet add mushrooms, carrots, rice, broth mix, 2 cups water, seasoning and salt substitute to taste. Place chicken on top of mixture. Cover and simmer 35 minutes or till chicken and rice are done.

6 servings.
Calories per serving: Approx. 250

MAIN DISH CHICKEN and PASTA SALAD WITH FRUIT – Serves 4

This is a great main course for hot summer nights. Make it up ahead and store it in a covered bowl. Toss with dressing before serving.

3 whole boneless chicken breasts, cooked and chopped into bite-
    size pieces
2 cups seedless green grapes
1 cup snow peas
20 spinach leaves, torn into pieces
1 6-ounce jar marinated artichoke hearts with marinade
1 kiwi, peeled and sliced
1/2 large cucumber, sliced
1/4 cup raisins (optional)
1 green onion, chopped
1 cup no-oil or low-cal creamy Italian or Italina salad dressing

Combine all ingredients except for dressing in large bowl. Toss gently to mix. Pour dressing over salad and toss again to coat. Serve immediately or save, chill and serve later.

CHICKEN FAJITAS *

very good

cut chicken in strips then cook

 2 T. light soy sauce
 4 flour tortillas
 1 cup chicken, cooked, skinless, cut into strips (or frozen
         diced chicken meat)
 1/2 large onion, thinly sliced
 1/2 large green pepper, cut into strips
 Salsa (homemade or prepared)
 1/8 t. cumin
 Dash hot pepper sauce, optional
 1 cup shredded lettuce
 Mock Sour Cream (see SAUCES), optional

To a Teflon skillet sprayed with non-stick coating add 1 T. soy sauce. Heat
to medium. Add onions and peppers and cook, stirring frequently. Lower
heat to low after 3 minutes and continue cooking till veggies are tender.
Add chicken, cumin and remaining soy sauce then heat through, stirring occasionally.

Heat flour tortillas on covered plate in microwave on High for 30 seconds or
wrapped in foil in the oven at 350 degrees for 10 minutes. Put tortilla on
a plate, fill with 1/4 of the chicken mixture, sprinkle with Salsa and
shredded lettuce, hot pepper sauce and Mock Sour Cream, if desired, roll up
and eat.

Serves 2 - 2 fajitas apiece, or 4 with one apiece.

* 1 cup imitation crabmeat or small cooked shrimp can be substituted for the
chicken.

NOTE: Be sure to check labels when purchasing Salsa if you choose not to
make your own. Many products contain more sugars, oils and salt than necessary. OLD EL PASO is a good one, although it contains some salt.

CHICKEN KABOBS — 2-3 servings

1 lb. boned, skinned chicken breasts, cut into 1-1/2" pieces
1 green bell pepper, cut into large chunks
2 small onions, quartered
Cherry tomatoes
Bottled no-oil vinaigrette or Italian dressing

Marinate the chicken and vegetable chunks (except cherry tomatoes) in the dressing for at least 1 hour. Drain. Alternate chicken, veggies and tomatoes on skewers. Broil in oven for about 20 minutes, turning every 5 minutes.

CORNY CHICKEN AND RICE

4 chicken pieces (thigh, leg or breast), skinned
2 packets chicken broth mix dissolved in 2-1/2 cups hot water
1 cup brown rice
1 cup sliced fresh mushrooms
1 cup chopped onion
1 clove garlic, minced
1 28-ounce can whole tomatoes, broken up, not drained
1 cup frozen corn
1 T. chopped pimiento
1/4 t. pepper and salt substitute

Moisten chicken with a bit of the prepared broth. Brown in broiler on each side, brushing with water or broth as they brown. Remove chicken when browned and arrange in casserole dish.

Preheat oven to 350 degrees.

In large saucepan combine rice, mushrooms, onion and garlic in 1/4 cup of the prepared broth. Cook over medium heat for 5 minutes. Add remainder of broth and bring to a boil. Cover, lower heat and simmer for 20 minutes. Add tomatoes, pimiento, corn and seasonings. Heat to boiling point. Pour over chicken in casserole. Cover and bake for 50 minutes. Uncover and cook 10 more minutes.

This dish can be prepared the day before, then put in the oven to cook 50 minutes before dinnertime.

CHICKEN BURGERS – 2 servings

      1 pound ground chicken (or grind your own from skinless, boned
            chicken breasts)
      1 clove garlic, minced
      1/8 cup onion, finely chopped
      1/2 t. salt substitute
      1/4 t. pepper

Mix all ingredients together. Form into 4 patties, each about 1/2" thick.
Wrap 2 in plastic and either freeze or save in refrigerator to use the next
day. On a grill pan sprayed with non-stick coating, broil the other 2
patties 6" from heat, for about 4 minutes on each side.

Serve with Homemade Catsup (see SAUCES)

If you're in the maintenance stage of your diet, eat the burger open-face on
a sourdough bun with lettuce and tomato.

PICADILLO – 6 servings

This is a strong-flavored Mexican stew.

      1 pound ground chicken
      1/8 t. garlic powder
      1 cup chopped onion
      1/2 t. dried cilantro leaves, crushed
      1/2 t. ground cinnamon
      1/4 t. salt and pepper
      1/8 t. each ground cloves and cumin
      1 medium-sized apple, pared and diced
      1 16-ounce can stewed tomatoes
      1/4 cup canned green chili peppers, chopped
      2 T. raisins

In Teflon skillet sprayed with non-stick coating add ground chicken, garlic,
onion and cilantro. Mix and stir till well blended and lightly browned.
Add remaining ingredients. Bring to a boil. Reduce heat to low and simmer
for 30 minutes.

Serve over a bed of steamed rice or roll up in a flour tortilla.

QUICK CHICKEN GOULASH

This is a real quick main dish. You can prepare it a day ahead and refrigerate it. Then reheat for serving.

>   1/2 lb. ground chicken
>   1 small onion, chopped
>   8 ounces elbow macaroni, cooked according to directions
>   1 cup Homemade Tomato Sauce (see SAUCES)
>   1 small can stewed tomatoes
>   1 package frozen corn, thawed
>   1 package frozen peas, thawed
>   1 t. mixed seasoning shake

In skillet sprayed with non-stick coating, break up and cook ground chicken and chopped onions till chicken is cooked through and onions are tender. Add remainder of ingredients and cook till heated through. Serve.

Serves 2-4 with leftovers.

EVEN QUICKER CHICKEN GOULASH - 4-6 servings

>   8 ounces ground chicken
>   1/2 onion, finely chopped
>   2 small cans tomato paste
>   1/4 cup water
>   2 cans Lite Veg-all (mixed vegetables)
>   2 t. Parsley Patch all-purpose blend
>   1/4 t. garlic powder
>   1/8 t. pepper
>   4 cups instant rice, cooked

In Teflon skillet sprayed with non-stick coating, cook chicken burger and onion till browned and cooked through. Add tomato paste and water, then mix well. Add seasonings; mix well. Add vegetables; mix well. Heat through and serve hot on bed of cooked rice.

SUPER QUICK APPLE ONION CHICKEN – Serves 2

Good with a side dish of acorn squash.

      1 T. apple juice
      1 onion, thinly sliced
      1/4 t. cinnamon
      1/8 t. coriander
      1/8 t. tumeric
      1/16 t. ground cloves
      2 boned, skinned chicken breasts halves (1 whole), cut into small thin slices
      2 small apples, peeled, cored and thinly sliced

In a Teflon fry pan, sprayed with non-stick coating, cook onion slices in apple juice over medium to high heat for 20 seconds. Add spices and cook for 15 seconds longer. Add chicken and cook for 3 minutes, stirring and turning pieces to cook evenly. Add apples and fry 2 minutes longer, stirring gently. Serve hot.

CHICKEN WITH A SPANISH FLAIR – Serves 2

This dish is great served over a bed of hot white rice.

      1 T. tomato paste mixed in 1/8 cup water
      1 small onion, finely chopped
      1/8 t. ground bay leaf
      1/8 t. tumeric
      1/16 t. ground cloves
      2 boned, skinned chicken breast halves (1 whole), cut into small thin slices
      3 scallions, cut into short strips
      2 small tomatoes, seeded and chopped, seasoned with 1/8 t. salt substitute

In a 12-inch skillet over medium to high heat, cook onion in tomato paste mixture for 2 minutes. Add chicken and cook for 2 more minutes, stirring to cook evenly. Add scallions and cook 1 more minute. Add tomatoes and cook minutes longer, stirring. Serve hot.

CHICKEN AND HERBS – Serves 2

This is another meal that goes great over hot rice. Try brown or wild rice to make it even more special. Using fresh herbs will also help make this a special treat.

                1 ounce dry white wine (or water if you choose not to use wine)
                1 garlic clove, minced
                2 t. chopped chives or onion greens
                1/2 t. parsley
                1/2 t. basil
                1/4 t. oregano
                1/8 t. ground bay leaf
                2 boned, skinned chicken breast halves (1 whole), cut into small
                     thin slices

In 10-inch fry pan, place wine, garlic, chives and herbs. Cook over medium to high heat for a few seconds, stirring. Add chicken and cook for 5 minutes, tossing pieces to cook evenly. Serve hot.

SPICEY CHICKEN – Serves 2

Cook some rice in chicken broth adding 1 T. raisins before cooking. It will give this meal an East Indian flair.

                1/2 t. cinnamon
                1/4 t. nutmeg
                1/4 t. tumeric
                1/8 t. ground cloves
                1 garlic clove, minced
                1/2 cup minced onion
                2 boned, skinned chicken breast halves, cut into small thin slices
                1/2 packet chicken broth mix dissolved in 1/2 cup hot water
                2 t. cornstarch blended with 1 ounce dry white wine (or water if
                     preferred)

In Teflon skillet, sprayed with non-stick coating, fry spices, garlic and onion over medium heat for 30 seconds. (Add droplets of water if veggies begin to stick.) Add chicken and fry 3 minutes more, stirring and tossing to cook evenly. Add broth mix and cook, covered, 1 minute. Add cornstarch and wine mixture and stir in quickly to blend and thicken. Serve hot.

HERBED CHICKEN A LA MICROWAVE

This chicken will have a creamy sauce. Serve it over cooked eggless pasta of your choice. Spinach pasta gives this dish a nice contrast in color. Serve with Stuffed Tomato Salad (see SALADS) for a very attractive meal. You won't believe you're on a diet.

> 2 boned, skinned chicken breast halves (1 whole)
> Paprika
> 1/2 cup fresh mushrooms, sliced
> 1 clove garlic, minced
> 1 T. water
> 2 t. cornstarch
> 1/2 packet chicken broth mix
> 1/2 cup warm water
> 1 t. cider vinegar
> 1 - 2 t. minced fresh tarragon leaves (or 1/4 t. dried)

Place chicken breast halves in microwaveable dish, with thicker parts toward outside. Sprinkle with paprika and cover with waxed paper. Microcook on Medium–High (70 % power) 7–9 minutes or till chicken is tender and no longer pink. Drain juices and set aside.

Combine mushrooms, garlic and 1 T. water in glass measure. Microcook on High, uncovered, 2 to 2-1/2 minutes, till mushrooms are tender, stirring once.

Combine cornstarch and dry broth mix; stir in hot water and vinegar until smooth. Add tarragon and stir into mushroom mixture. Microcook on High, uncovered, 2 to 2-1/2 minutes, or until mixture boils and thickens, stirring once.

Spoon sauce over chicken. Microcook on High, uncovered 1 to 1-1/2 minutes longer, till heated through.

Serves 2.

CHICKEN TERIYAKI – 2 servings

Serve over cooked white rice with a side dish of Sweet and Sour Vegetables (see VEGETABLES) for an oriental dinner.

        2 boned, skinned chicken breast halves, cut into small thin slices
        1/4 cup light soy sauce
        1/2 packet chicken broth mix dissolved in 1/3 cup warm water
        2 t. cornstarch

Combine chicken pieces and soy in a 1–quart microwaveable casserole. Cover with plastic wrap and refrigerate at least 20 minutes to marinate. Drain marinade and reserve. Recover chicken with plastic wrap, venting one corner. Microcook on High 3 minutes; pour off juices.

Gradually stir chicken broth into cornstarch in small bowl. Add reserved marinade and blend. Stir mixture into chicken. Microcook on High 2 to 2-1/2 minutes, or until thickened, stirring once or twice. Let stand, covered, for 2 minutes to complete cooking. Serve.

OATMEAL BAKED CHICKEN WITH LEMON

        1-1/4 cups quick or old fashioned uncooked oats
        2 T. chopped fresh parsley (or 1 T. dry parsley flakes)
        1 clove garlic, minced (or 1/8 t. garlic powder)
        2-1/2 to 3 pound broiler fryer chicken, cut up and skinned
        1/2 cup low fat milk (or more as needed)
        Lemon wedges

Preheat oven to 375 degrees. Process oats in blender or food processor about 1 minute. Add parsley and garlic; stir to blend. Coat chicken pieces in seasoned oats; dip into milk; coat again with seasoned oats. Place on baking sheet sprayed with non–stick coating. Bake 55–60 minutes or until juices run clear when chicken is pricked with fork. Squeeze lemon over chicken just before serving.

4 servings.

NOTES
=======

FISH and SEAFOOD DISHES

=================================

SHRIMP

These cook up so well in a microwave oven . . .

> 1/2 lb. medium shrimp, peeled and deveined

Arrange around the edge of a glass pie plate, tails toward the center. Cover. Cook on High 2-3 minutes. Serve on a bed of white steamed rice, sprinkled with a paprika, chili powder mixture. Or chill and serve with cocktail sauce.*

2 servings.

Calories per serving (shrimp only): Approx. 100

* To Homemade Catsup (see SAUCES) add 1/4 t. horseradish (not creamed)

FISH

Any kind of fish steak or fillet can be broiled or baked. Instead of butter sauces use a sprinkling of lemon juice and any of the following herbs or spices:

> onion powder
> pepper
> thyme
> paprika
> onion powder
> dillweed
> parsley
> basil

Depending on the thickness of the fish, broil 10 minutes on each side (6" from heat). Or bake at 350 degree about 25 minutes.

FISH FILLET BAKE

2 fish fillets (about 3 ounces each)
White pepper
Paprika
1/2 cup chopped onion
1/8 t. black pepper
1 T. chopped parsley
1/4 t. basil
1/4 t. thyme
4 t. lemon juice

Sprinkle fillets with dash of white pepper and paprika. Place in a flat casserole dish or individual ramekins. Combine remaining ingredients in small pan. Add 1/2 cup water and bring to a boil. Pour over fish and bake at 350 degrees for 25 minutes.

Serves 2.

CREOLE FISH FILLETS

1 pound fish fillets
1/2 cup chopped onion
1/2 cup chopped celery
1/4 cup chopped green pepper
1 packet sugar substitute
1/2 t. oregano leaves
1/8 t. pepper
1 8-ounce can (1 cup) stewed tomatoes, undrained, cut up
Dash hot pepper sauce

Heat oven to 350 degrees. Arrange fish fillets in 12" x 8" or 8" square baking dish. Spray with non-stick coating.

In Teflon skillet sprayed with non-stick coating, cook onion, celery and pepper in 1/4 cup of the stewed tomato juices over medium-low heat, covered, till tender. Stir in remaining ingredients. Spoon mixture over fish. Bake for 15-20 minutes.

4 servings.

Calories per serving: Approx. 120

POACHED SALMON AND VEGGIES

> 2 salmon steaks (1" thick)
> 2 T. lemon juice
> 1 carrot, sliced
> 1/3 medium onion, sliced
> 1 stalk celery, sliced
> 1/2 medium zucchini, sliced
> 1/2 t. no-salt mixed seasonings
> Bay leaf

Arrange salmon steaks in non-stick skillet. Pour lemon juice over them and fill the skillet with 1" water. Add remaining ingredients, except zucchini. Bring to a boil, then reduce heat and cover. Simmer the fish and veggies for 15 minutes. Add zucchini and cook for 5 minutes more or until salmon flakes with a fork. Transfer salmon and veggies to serving platter, remove bay leaf and serve hot.

This dish is also very good served over a bed of steamed rice.

Serves 2.

SPICY BRAISED HALIBUT STEAKS - 2 servings

> 2 10-ounce halibut steaks
> 2 T. light soy sauce
> 1 ripe tomato, chopped
> 1/2 green pepper, chopped
> 1 small onion, chopped
> 1/2 t. chili powder
> 1 clove garlic, minced
> 1/4 t. salt substitute
> Dash crushed hot red pepper

In a large skillet place soy sauce. Add remaining ingredients, except fish. Bring to a boil. Add halibut steaks. Cover and simmer on low 4-6 minutes per 1/2" thickness. Transfer fish to serving plates. Spoon vegetables over fish.

Try serving this fish with a baked potato and spoon some of the vegetable mixture into the potato.

FAKE CRAB CASSEROLE

This delicious dish should take no more than 10 minutes to prepare. It is so good you feel like you're cheating. Try serving it with a tomato salad or with stewed tomatoes.

2 T. light soy sauce
1/2 cup chopped onion
1 12–ounce package imitation crab meat, thawed if frozen
1 t. no–salt Parsley Patch mixed seasoning shake or other
      brand
2 cups rice, cooked
1 cup peas, canned, or frozen (thawed)

In a Teflon skillet sprayed with non–stick coating, add the soy sauce and onions then cook, covered, for 5 minutes. Add the seasoning and crab-meat then cook another 3 minutes. Add the rice and peas then cook, covered, stirring occasionally, until heated through and peas are cooked. Serve.

Serves 2 with leftovers.

SALMON BUNDLES

This is a fast dish that uses your magical microwave oven.

2 T. carrots, julienned
2 T. celery, julienned
2 6–ounce salmon fillets, 1/2" thick
2 T. tomatoes, diced
1 t. parsley, minced
2 t. white wine (optional)
2 t. lemon juice
black pepper to taste

Spread out two 12" square pieces of plastic wrap. Divide evenly and arrange carrots and celery in the centers. Lay salmon on top of the vegetables. Top with the remaining ingredients divided evenly. Seal packages and cook on High for 2 to 2-1/2 minutes.

Serves 2.

A DILLY OF A FISH DISH

1/2 t. dillweed, crushed
1/4 t. parsley
1/8 t. thyme
Few drops lemon juice
1 pound thin fish fillets
3 ounces dry white wine, hot
1 t. cornstarch blended with 2 T. skim milk

In 12-inch Teflon skillet, sprayed with non-stick coating, place lemon juice and herbs and cook over medium heat for a few seconds, stirring. Add fish fillets and cook 1 minute, without turning. Turn fish and add wine. Cook 2 minutes more. Transfer fillets to plate. Add cornstarch and milk mixture then stir into pan juice quickly to blend and thicken. Place fillets back in pan and cook 30 seconds more or till heated through.

2 servings.

CLASSIC SALMON LOAF

1/2 cup cracker crumbs (put unsalted fat-free crackers in blender
        or processor)
2-1/2 cups cooked, flaked salmon
1/3 cup chopped green onion
1/2 cup finely chopped celery
Juice of 1/2 lemon
1 t. salt substitute
1/2 t. pepper
2 egg whites
1/2 cup lite mayonnaise

Preheat oven to 375 degrees.

Mix all ingredients together. Pack into a loaf pan sprayed with non-stick coating and bake for 30-45 minutes until firm and browned on top.

4-6 servings.

CRABCAKES

1 pound crabmeat, or imitation crabmeat
1/4 cup finely chopped onion
2 egg whites
1 T. mustard
1 T. lite (low fat) mayonnaise
1 t. lemon juice
1/2 cup cracker crumbs (or day old sourdough bread crumbs)
3 T. finely chopped fresh parsley
1/2 t. Worcestershire Sauce

Combine all ingredients. Form into patties. Place on baking pan sprayed with non-stick coating. Broil till golden brown on each side.

2 servings.

ORANGE-SAUCED HALIBUT

1 pound fresh or frozen halibut steaks, thawed
2 t. cornstarch
1/2 packet chicken broth mix
2 T. thinly sliced green onion
2/3 cup orange juice
1 orange, peeled and sliced; each slice cut into quarters

Preheat oven to 450 degrees.

Place halibut in a baking dish. For sauce, in small saucepan stir together cornstarch, broth mix, onion and orange juice. Cook and stir till thickened and bubbly. Stir orange pieces into juice mixture. Pour over fish. Bake for 10-12 minutes or till fish flakes easily with a fork.

4 servings.

NOTES
======

DESSERTS YOU DESERVE

The chapter on desserts is relatively small, because once you've developed a taste for good, healthy foods and are allowed to eat as many vegggies as you want, or have snacks like Rye Krisps and are eating meals of good, healthy, filling soups and casseroles, you should find that you have little room left for desserts, and that your desire for them has diminished.

The craving of sweets is partially a result of low blood sugar. If you eat a well-balanced diet your blood sugar will not experience such extreme highs and lows.

The desserts listed are mostly fruit desserts. Any kind of fresh fruit is allowed on this diet, just keep the calorie count in mind because they do add up, even though they are healthy calories. Finish a meal with a crisp apple, a bowl of strawberries or a slice of melon. You will find they satisfy your sweet cravings and remove the temptation to eat some simple sugar-type dessert.

There are some diet dessert products on the market, so check out your grocery store. Weight Watchers makes a low-cal pudding (use nonfat or skim milk) and there are many gelatin dessert products with very few calories. Batterlite Whitlock puts out a Lite Whip Mousse but it contains some sugar so don't use any until you are on a weight control maintenance program, then limit your useage.

BAKED APPLES – 4 servings (approx. 50 calories each)

>   2 apples, cored, cut in half
>   1/2 t. cinnamon
>   2 t. raisins

Preheat oven to 400 degrees.

Place apple halves in baking dish, cut sides down. Cover with 1/2 cup water. Bake for 20 minutes.

Remove, turn over and sprinkle evenly with cinnamon. Place 1/2 t. raisins in center of each half. Return to oven for 5 more minutes.

SPICED GRAPEFRUIT

Double this recipe and make a big batch of these delicious grapefruit sections to have on hand. They are especially good as your fruit choice at breakfast.

> 2 medium grapefruit
> Unsweetened grapefruit juice
> Artificial sweetener equivalent to 2 t. sugar
> 2 T. white wine vinegar
> 1/2 t. whole cloves
> 2 3-inch sticks of cinnamon

Peel and section grapefruits over bowl, saving juice and membranes. Set sections aside. Squeeze membranes to extract juice and throw membranes away. Measure reserved juice. Add grapefruit juice to equal 3/4 cup.

Combine juice, sugar, vinegar, cloves, cinnamon in saucepan (NOT ALUM-INUM). Bring to a boil, stirring constantly. Reduce heat and simmer 10 minutes. Remove from heat. Cool.

Strain and discard spices. Pour juice over grapefruit sections. Cover and chill at least 8 hours.

3 servings. Calories per serving: Approx. 90

SPICED PINEAPPLE – Serves 2

> 1 20-ounce can pineapple chunks in their own juice, drained*
> 1 t. brown sugar
> 1/8 t. each cinnamon, nutmeg and allspice
> 1 T. lime peel

Place pineapple in microwaveable dish. Cover with plastic wrap and microcook on High 3-4 minutes. Combine brown sugar and spices, then sprinkle over the pineapple. Stir and cook 1-2 minutes more, till sugar is just melted. Sprinkle with lime peelings.

* Or substitute 1 small fresh pineapple. Peel, core and cut in 1/2" chunks.

FRUITED YOGURT

Make this a special dessert by serving it in a champagne flute or wine glass.

> 2 cups plain, low fat yogurt
> 2 cups fruit: Your choice of one or a combination of:
>
>> sliced strawberries, blackberries
>> blueberries, huckleberries
>> raspberries, or other bush berries
>> water-packed, canned cherries, halved

Stir fruit into the yogurt, breaking some of it to color the yogurt. Chill till serving time.

4 servings.

NOTE: You may also stir in 1 or 2 drops of vanilla, almond or rum extract for some flavoring variety.

PINEAPPLE ICE

> 1 20-ounce can pineapple chunks in their own juice,
>> drained (reserve 3/4 cup of the juice)
> 1/4 cup skim milk

Spread pineapple chunks on baking sheet. Make sure they are not touching each other. Freeze chunks until hard. Drop into blender or food processor. Add milk and reserved pineapple juice. Process about 20 seconds or till mixture is smooth.

Serve immediately or spoon into container, cover tightly and freeze for serving latter. Keeps at least 1 week.

Makes 2-1/2 cups.

Calories per 1/2 cup serving: Approx. 80

APPLE/PINEAPPLE PUDDING

This takes some time to make but will last several days in the refrigerator and is a very satisfying dessert. Serve it with a dollop of Mock Sour Cream or plain, lowfat yogurt.

> 1-1/2 cups all-purpose flour
> 2 cups nonfat milk
> 1 20-ounce can pineapple chunks in their own juice, drained, reserve juice (Add water to liquid to equal 1/4 cup if needed)
> 2 t. vanilla extract
> 4 egg whites
> 4 apples, peeled, cored and sliced
> 1 t. ground cinnamon
> 1/4 t. ginger
> 1/8 t. nutmeg

Preheat oven to 400 degrees. Combine flour, milk, 1/4 cup of the reserved pineapple juice and vanilla. Beat egg whites till frothy with a fork. Add to flour mixture and mix well. Spread apple slices on bottom of an 8" x 12" non-stick baking dish. Sprinkle pineapple chunks over apples. Mix together cinnamon, ginger and nutmeg. Sprinkle half of spice mixture over the fruit. Mix the rest into the batter. Pour batter over the fruit. Bake 30 minutes or till lightly browned and well set. Cut into squares to serve.

MIXED BERRIES WITH RICOTTA – 6 servings

> 1 pint fresh raspberries (or frozen with no added sugar, thawed and drained)
> 1 pint fresh blackberries, boysenberries or blueberries (or frozen with no added sugar, thawed and drained)
> 1 container (15-16 ounces) low fat ricotta cheese
> 2-3 T. low fat milk
> 1 t. vanilla
> 1 t. granulated artificial sweetener

Combine berries in large bowl. Sprinkle with granulated artificial sweetener, if desired. Cover and refrigerate. In processor or mixing bowl blend cheese, milk, vanilla and 1 t. artificial sweetener till smooth and creamy. Serve a dollop of blended mixture on top of a bowl of the berries.

BERRY FOOL

This is a traditional English dessert which normally uses whipping cream. We will substitute low fat yogurt for the cream in this recipe to make it just as delicious but much lower in calories and healthier for you.

> 1 pint each fresh blueberries and blackberries, cleaned
> 1 t. granulated sugar substitute
> 1/2 t. rum, vanilla or almond extract
> 1/2 t. cinnamon
> 1/4 cup plus 1 T. cold water
> 2 t. cornstarch
> 1 pint low fat vanilla yogurt

Place half of the berries in a medium saucepan with sugar substitute, extract, cinnamon and 1/4 cup cold water. Cover and bring to boil over medium heat, stirring occasionally.

Meanwhile, stir together the cornstarch and remaining 1 T. cold water in a small bowl, forming a smooth paste. Add this mixture to the boiling fruit and cook, uncovered, stirring constantly, for 2 minutes or until the berry mixture has thickened slightly. Remove from heat and immediately place a piece of plastic wrap on the surface of the cooked berry mixture to prevent formation of a skin. Cool the mixture completely.

Stir the remaining berries into the cooked and cooled mixture. Stir yogurt in its container until smooth. Spoon berry mixture into parfait glass or champagne flutes, layer with dollops of yogurt. Alternate layers ending with a berry layer and a small dollop of yogurt. Refrigerate till serving time.

6 servings.

APPLE–PEAR CRISP

1 cup rolled oats
1 cup wheat flour
1/2 cup Grape Nuts cereal
2 t. cinnamon
1/4 t. nutmeg
2 cups unsweetened apple juice
1 cup sliced apples
1 cup sliced pears
1/4 cup raisins
1 T. lemon juice
2 t. cornstarch

Preheat oven to 350 degrees.

For CRUST: Combine oats, flour, cereal, 1 t. of the cinnamon and nut-meg. Stir in 1 cup of the apple juice till mixture holds together. Press half of the mixture over bottom and up sides of a non–stick 9" pie pan. (Or spray with non–stick coating.) Bake for 5 minutes. Save remaining mixture for the top.

FILLING: Combine apples, pears, remaining 1 cup of apple juice, raisins, remaining 2 t. of cinnamon, lemon juice and cornstarch in a medium saucepan. Bring to a boil, then reduce heat and simmer about 10 minutes or until apples and pears are slightly tender. Remove apples, pears and raisins with a slotted spoon and place in cooked pie shell. Increase heat and continue cooking sauce till it thickens. Pour sauce over apples, pears and raisins. Crumble remaining crust mixture over the top. Raise oven heat to 375 degrees and bake for 30 minutes.

Serve warm with a dollop of Mock Sour Cream or low fat yogurt.

6–8 servings.

NOTE: You may use 2 cups of apples and leave out the pears if desired.

NOTES

SNACKS

POPCORN

Use an air popper or microwave oven to pop your corn and leave off the butter and salt. It may taste bland at first, but once the pounds start to drop off, you should see this snack in a different light. Use popcorn to fill in those "desperate" times when you just HAVE to have something to eat . . . when the growlies really get to you.

If you must, sprinkle a bit of salt substitute on the popcorn. Other sprinkles that satisfy: garlic powder, onion powder or chili powder.

ENJOY!!!

TORTILLA CHIPS

1 package flour or corn tortillas, cut into quarters

Lay the quarters on a non-stick baking sheet. Do not overlap. Sprinkle with one of the following seasonings:

> salt substitute
> onion powder
> garlic powder
> chili powder
> cumin
> paprika

Bake at 400 degrees until crisp and beginning to brown. Check often.

Serve with Salsa (see SAUCES), Green Pea Gaucamole*, PACE Picante Sauce, Bean Dip* or Mock Sour Cream (see SAUCES).

* Recipes will follow.

BEAN DIP

1 can pinto beans, drained and mashed.

Choose any of the following to be added for flavor:

> onion powder
> garlic powder
> diced green chilies
> chili powder
> small tomato, chopped
> Dash of hot pepper sauce
> ground cumin

Blend well. Serve hot or cold with tortilla chips.

Makes about 1 cup.

GREEN PEA GUACAMOLE

> 2 cups cooked green peas, drained and chilled
> 1 4–ounce can diced green chili peppers, rinsed
> 2 T. chopped onion
> 2 T. lime juice
> 1 clove garlic, minced
> Few dashes hot pepper sauce

In a blender or food processor combine all ingredients. Cover and blend or process till smooth. Cover and chill till serving time.

Makes 1–2/3 cups

6 servings.

Calories per serving: Approx. 50

MOCK POTATO CHIPS

Early in the day or on the day before, wash and dry potatoes. Drop, un-peeled, into boiling water. Lower heat and simmer till they are just barely tender. Drain off water and refrigerate.

When cold, slice into rounds. DO NOT PEEL. Spread rounds on a non-stick baking sheet. (Or spray a regular baking sheet with non-stick coating.)

Season with one or a combination of the following:

> salt substitute
> onion powder
> garlic powder
> no-salt seasoning mix
> chili powder
> ground black pepper

Bake in 400 degree oven till browned. Flip over and cook till browned again. The chips will be crispy and satisfying.

Serve plain or with Salsa (see SAUCES), Onion Dip*, Clam Dip*, or Herbed Curry Yogurt Dip*.

Calories vary: 1 small potato contains about 75 calories and is equivalent to about 9 slices.

* Recipes to follow.

ONION DIP

> 1 cup Mock Sour Cream (see SAUCES)
> 2 T. onion flakes, toasted in oven till browned

Mix together. Serve with raw veggies or Mock Potato Chips.

CLAM DIP

1 cup Mock Sour Cream (see SAUCES)
1/2 cup canned, chopped clams, drained well
1/2 t. lemon juice
1/4 t. Worcestershire Sauce

Mix together and serve with raw veggies or Mock Potato Chips.

HERBED CURRY YOGURT DIP

1/2 cup plain low fat yogurt
1/2 cup Mock Sour Cream (see SAUCES)
2 T. Homemade Catsup (see SAUCES)
1/8 t. chili powder
2 t. vinegar
1 t. curry powder
1/2 t. onion powder
1/2 t. dried thyme, crushed
1/4 t. salt substitute, optional
1/8 t. pepper

Combine all ingredients in bowl. Cover and refrigerate till serving time.
Serve with raw veggies or Mock Potato Chips.

Makes 1–1/4 cups dip.

NOTE: You may delete the salt substitute and add 6 ounces of imitation
crabmeat, chopped, for a crabmeat currried yogurt dip. Yield is 1–3/4
cups dip.

PITA TOASTS

These are good not only as a snack, but as an appetizer or meal accompaniment. In summer serve pita toast snacks with Gazpacho (see SOUPS) for a light Mexican luncheon.

TOASTED PITAS

Cut one large Pita bread pocket into 6 triangles. Pull each triangle apart to make 2. (Total chips = 12) Place on cookie sheet in 350 degree oven and toast, rough side up, for 5 minutes.

Sprinkle with any of the following before or after toasting:

> salt substitute
> oregano
> basil
> chili powder
> pepper
> paprika
> other spices of your choice

NOTE: Sprinkling the toasts with cinnamon and sugar substitute makes a good breakfast "cracker" or after meals "cookie".

OTHER TOPPINGS FOR TOASTED PITA TRIANGLES:

-- place 1/2 t. catsup, dash of tabasco and sprinkling of oregano on each triangle before toasting. Makes a pizza-like snack.

-- place a tomato wedge on each triangle and sprinkle with chopped scallions before toasting.

-- place 1/2 t. Homemade Catsup mixed with a dash of horseradish (not creamed) on each toast AFTER toasting and then place 1 medium deveined, cooked shrimp on top of the sauce.

ORANGEY CHICKEN WINGS – 16 to 18 servings

This is a good snack to fix for a crowd. Prepare the wings a day ahead and cook when needed.

> 1-1/2 lbs. chicken wings, skinned, rinsed and wing tips removed
> 2 T. light soy sauce
> 2/3 cup orange juice
> 1 T. dry sherry, optional
> 1 T. cornstarch
> 1/4 t. ground ginger
> 1/8 t. aniseed
> Dash ground red pepper
> Dash ground cloves

Cut each wing at joint to make 2 sections. In a 12"x7-1/2"x2" microwaveable baking dish, arrange chicken pieces with meaty portions toward edge of dish. Brush chicken with 1 T. of the light soy sauce. Cover with waxed paper and microcook on High 6 minutes, turning dish a half-turn once. Drain well.

Meanwhile, in a 2-cup glass measure, combine orange juice, sherry, 1 T. light soy sauce, cornstarch, ginger, aniseed, pepper and cloves. After wings are cooked, microcook sauce, uncovered, on High 3-5 minutes or till thickened and bubbly, stirring every minute till thickened, then stirring every 30 seconds. Pour thickened liquid over chicken.* Cook, covered, on High 3-5 minutes or till chicken is no longer pink. Serve warm.

16-18 servings.

* Before covering the chicken with the sauce you can refrigerate it and finish cooking the required time a day later.

SHRIMP AND FRUIT KABOBS – 30 servings

Another crowd pleaser!

> 1 8–ounce package frozen shrimp, peeled and deveined, thawed
> 1 8–1/4–ounce can pineapple chunks in their own juice, drain-
> ed; reserve juice
> 1 medium apple, cut into 1" pieces
> 1/4 cup DIET orange marmalade
> 2 t. light soy sauce
> 1 t. cornstarch

In a 1–quart casserole, microcook shrimp on High 1 minute. On wooden toothpicks, thread 1 shrimp and either a pineapple or apple chunk. Arrange kabobs in a 12"x8"x2" casserole. Set aside.

For glaze, in a 2–cup glass measure, combine 4 T. of the reserved pineap- ple juice with, marmalade, soy sauce and cornstarch. Microcook, un- covered, on High 2–3 minutes or till thickened and bubbly, stirring every 30 seconds. Brush glaze on kabobs. Cover with vented clear plastic wrap. Microcook on High 3–5 minutes or till shrimp turn pink. Rear- range, turn over and brush with glaze once during cooking.

SALMON STEAK TARTARE

> 1 lb. very fresh salmon, chopped fine
> 4 T. capers, drained, rinsed and chopped
> 1 t. lemon juice
> 2 T. salt-free Dijon mustard with herbs
> 2 T. chopped fresh parsley
> 2 new potatoes (6–ounce size), boiled, cooled, peeled and diced
> 3 small beets, baked or boiled, cooled, peeled and diced
> 4 T. finely chopped red onion

Mix salmon, capers, lemon juice, mustard and parsley together. Chill to blend flavors.

To serve: Arrange salmon mixture in a mound (on plate covered with red lettuce if desired). Garnish with rows or small mounds of potatoes, beets and onions. Serve with sliced sourdough baguettes or pita bread cut into wedges.

NOTES

SAMPLE OF MENUS

All dishes mentioned in this chapter have recipes included in this book or on the snack sheet. For each day of the week you will find an eye-opening breakfast, a luscious lunch and a dinner well worth coming home for. Measurements are not included. Remember, you're on a diet, and while these are all low fat, low sodium, low sugar and low cholesterol foods and recipes, it doesn't mean you can "pig out" and expect to lose weight. Use your common sense. Most recipes give the serving amounts – eat only one serving.

You may find that you can't comfortably eat all of your meal. Rather than stuffing yourself and feeling uncomfortable, save parts of the meal for a snack to be eaten later in the day or evening.

Another surprising and welcome aspect of this diet is that after a meal you will find you are less likely to get sleepy. As you know, people often feel they need a nap soon after eating. By way of simplification, think of it as though an extra portion of your blood has left the brain to go down and help with the job of digesting all that food you ate. Lighter meals with fewer calories means a LIVELIER YOU !

MONDAY

Breakfast:

Hot oatmeal, with 1/4 t. cinnamon and 1 t. raisins
Nonfat milk
Hot Sliced Apples

Lunch:

Cup of Cream of Broccoli Soup
Small green salad with sliced cucumber and a small
      tomato, cut up
No-oil salad dressing of your choice
2 Rye Krisps or Rice Cakes
1 small apple

Dinner:

Broiled Chicken
Twice-Baked Potato
Steamed asparagus sprinkled with butter substitute and
      tarragon
Pineapple Ice

TUESDAY

Breakfast: Bowl of Product 19 cold cereal with sliced banana
Nonfat milk
1/2 grapefruit

Lunch: Carrot Bisque
Chicken Fajitas made with flour tortillas
Homemade Salsa
Mock Sour Cream
Orange sections

Dinner: Steamed shrimp
Parslied Rice
Sweet and Sour Vegetables
Spiced Pineapple

WEDNESDAY

Breakfast: Scrambled Egg with onion and herbs
Sourdough toast with fruit spread
Spiced Grapefruit

Lunch: Whole wheat pita bread stuffed with chopped vegetables
and sprinkled with 1 t. diet dressing
Cup of Lentil Soup
Small bunch of grapes

Dinner: Spaghetti with Homemade Tomato Sauce and added ground
chicken
Green salad with no–oil salad dressing
Sourdough bread toast rubbed with garlic clove
Baked Apple Dessert

THURSDAY

Breakfast: Cottage Cheese Pancakes with fresh berries
and Mock Sour Cream
Unsweetened fruit juice

Lunch: Quick Turkey–Apple Salad
Cup of Onion Soup
Pita Toasts or Lavosh
Tangerine

Dinner: Chili Rice and Beans
Green Salad with no–oil salad dressing
Homemade Tortilla Chips with chili powder
Yogurt with dash of banana extract and blueberries

FRIDAY

Breakfast: Low–cal cranberry juice
French Toast with low–cal syrup
Low fat, plain yogurt with berries

Lunch: Bowl of Creamy Cauliflower Soup
Stuffed Tomato Salad
Norwegian flatbread
Spiced Pineapple

Dinner: Vegetable Enchiladas with
Mock Sour Cream
Homemade Tortilla Chips with
Green Pea Guacamole and
Homemade Salsa
Melon Balls or Slices of Melon

SATURDAY

Breakfast:
Strawberries with nonfat milk and sugar substitute
Scrambled Eggs with Tomato
Sourdough toast with spreadable fruit

Lunch:
Quick Vichyssoise
Chicken Salad with Grapes
Rye Krisps
Apple

Dinner:
Chinese Cole Slaw
Chinese Spaghetti
Pita toasts with sesame seeds
Plain low fat yogurt with drop of almond extract and
    sliced bananas

SUNDAY

Breakfast:
Potato Pancakes with Mock Sour Cream and
Homemade Applesauce
Grapefruit half broiled with dash of cinnamon and sugar
    substitute

Dinner:
Spicy Halibut Steaks
Artichoke with Homemade Mayonnaise
Tossed green salad with low-cal dressing
Apple/Pineapple Pudding with dollop of Mock Sour Cream

Supper:
Bowl of Any Day Vegetable Soup
Mock Potato Chips with
Clam Dip
Pineapple Ice

INDEX

INDEX OF RECIPES
==================

NOTES